SEEKING GOD'S BEST

Gospel Light is a Christian publisher dedicated to serving the local church. We believe God's vision for Gospel Light is to provide church leaders with biblical, user-friendly materials that will help them evangelize, disciple and minister to children, youth and families.

It is our prayer that this Gospel Light resource will help you discover biblical truth for your own life and help you minister to others. May God richly bless you.

For a free catalog of resources from Gospel Light, please contact your Christian supplier or contact us at 1-800-4-GOSPEL or www.gospellight.com.

PUBLISHING STAFF
William T. Greig, Chairman
Kyle Duncan, Publisher
Dr. Elmer L. Towns, Senior Consulting Publisher
Pam Weston, Senior Editor
Patti Pennington Virtue, Associate Editor
Jeff Kempton, Editorial Assistant
Hilary Young, Editorial Assistant
Bayard Taylor, M.Div., Senior Editor, Biblical and Theological Issues
Barbara LeVan Fisher, Packaging Concept and Design
Samantha A. Hsu, Cover and Internal Designer

ISBN 0-8307-2925-9
© 2002 First Place
All rights reserved.
Printed in the U.S.A.

CAUTION
The information contained in this book is intended to be solely informational and educational. It is assumed that the First Place participant will consult a medical or health professional before beginning this or any other weight-loss or physical fitness program.

CONTENTS

FOREWORD

My introduction to Bible study came when I joined First Place in March of 1981. I had been in church since I was a small child, but the extent of my study of the Bible had been reading my Sunday School quarterly on Saturday night. On Sunday morning, I would listen to my Sunday School teacher as she taught God's Word to me. During the worship service, I would listen to our pastor as he taught God's Word to me. Digging out the truths of the Bible for myself had frankly never entered my mind.

Perhaps you are right where I was back in 1981. If so, you are in for a blessing you never dreamed possible. As you start studying the truths of the Bible for yourself, you will see God begin to open your understanding of His Word. Bible study is one of the nine commitments of the First Place program. The First Place Bible studies are designed to be done on a daily basis. Each day's study will take approximately 15 to 20 minutes to complete, but you will be discovering the deep truths of God's Word as you work through each week's study.

There are many in-depth Bible studies on the market. The First Place Bible studies are not designed for the purpose of in-depth study. They are designed to be used in conjunction with the other eight commitments of the program to bring balance into our lives. Our desire is for each member to begin having a personal quiet time with God each day. This time alone with God would include a time of prayer, Bible reading and Bible study. Having a quiet time is a daily discipline that will bring the rich rewards of balance, something we all need.

A part of each week's study is the Bible memory verse for the week. You will find a CD at the back of this Bible study that contains all 10 of the memory verses for the study. The CD has an upbeat tempo suitable for use when exercising. The songs help you to easily memorize the verses and retain them for future reference. If you will memorize Scripture as you study, God will use His Word to transform your life.

Almost every First Place member I have talked with about the program says, "The weight loss is wonderful, but the most important thing I have received from my association with First Place is learning to study God's Word."

God bless you as you begin this exciting journey toward a balanced life. God will richly bless your efforts to give Him first place in your life. Remember Matthew 6:33: "But seek first his kingdom and his righteousness, and all these things will be given to you as well."

Carole Lewis
First Place National Director

INTRODUCTION

The First Place Bible studies were developed to be used in conjunction with the First Place weight-loss program. However, the studies could also be used by anyone desiring to learn more about God's Word and His will, with the added bonus of learning more about living a healthy lifestyle.

A Balanced Life

First Place is a Christ-centered health program, emphasizing balance in the physical, mental, emotional and spiritual areas of life. The First Place program is meant to be a daily process. As we learn to keep Christ first in our lives, we will find that He is the One who satisfies our hunger and our every need.

God's Word contains guidelines for maintaining our physical well-being, equipping us mentally to make right choices, providing emotional stability to handle everyday circumstances as well as crisis situations, and growing spiritually as we deepen our relationship with Him.

The Nine Commitments

The First Place program has nine commitments that will help you draw closer to the Lord and aid you in establishing a solid, consistent and more healthy Christian life. Each commitment is a necessary and important part of the goal of First Place to help you become healthier and stronger in all areas of your life—living the abundant life He has planned for each of us. To help you achieve growth in all four areas, First Place asks you to keep these nine commitments:

1. Attendance
2. Encouragement
3. Prayer
4. Bible Reading
5. Scripture Memory Verse
6. Bible Study
7. Live-It Plan
8. Commitment Record
9. Exercise

The Components

There are six distinct components to this Bible study to aid you in bringing balance to your life. These components include the 10-week Bible study, 6 Wellness Worksheets, 2 weeks of menu plans, the leader's discussion guide, 13 Commitment Records and the Scripture memory CD.

The Bible Study

Each week of each 10-week Bible study is divided into five daily assignments with Days 6 and 7 set aside for reflections on the week's lesson. The following guidelines will help make your study more enjoyable and profitable:

- Set aside 15 to 20 minutes each day to complete the daily assignment. It's best not to attempt to complete a week's worth of Bible study in one day.
- Pray before each day's study and ask God to give you understanding and a teachable heart.
- Keep in mind that the ultimate goal of Bible study is not for knowledge only but also for application and a changed life.
- First Place suggests using the New International Version of the Bible to complete the studies.
- Don't feel anxious if you can't seem to find the correct answer. Many times the Word will speak differently to different people, depending upon where they are in their walk with God and the season of life they are experiencing.
- Be prepared to discuss with your fellow First Place members what you learned that week through your study.

Wellness Worksheets

The informative and interactive Wellness Worksheets have been developed by Dr. Jody Wilkinson at the Cooper Institute in Dallas, Texas. These worksheets are intended to help you understand and achieve balance in all four areas of your life: physical, mental, emotional and spiritual. Your leader will assign specific worksheets as At-Home Assignments throughout the 13-week session.

Menu Plans

The two-week menu plans were developed especially for First Place by Chef Scott Wilson. Each menu is meant to simplify meal planning and include food exchanges. These meals are based on the MasterCook software that uses a database of over 6,000 food items, which was prepared using United States Department of Agriculture (USDA) publications and information from food manufacturers.

Leader's Discussion Guide

This discussion guide is provided to help the First Place leader guide a group through this Bible study. It provides information for the leader to prepare for each weekly group meeting.

Personal Weight Record

The Personal Weight Record is for the member to use to keep a record of weight loss. After the weigh-in at each week's meeting, the member will record any loss or gain on the chart.

Commitment Records

Thirteen Commitment Records (CRs) are provided in the back of this Bible study. For your convenience these have been printed on perforated paper so that you may easily remove them from the book and carry them with you through each week as you keep your First Place commitments. Directions for filling out the CRs precede those pages.

Scripture Memory CD

Since Scripture memory is such a vital part of the First Place program, the Scripture memory CD for this study is included in the back inside cover. The verses for this study are set to music that can be listened to as you work, play or travel. The CD can be an effective tool as you exercise since the first verse is set to music with a warm-up tempo, the next eight verses are set to workout tempo, and the music of the last verse can be used for a cooldown.

SEEKING GOD'S BEST

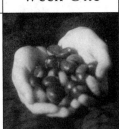

MEMORY VERSE

Then Jesus declared, "I am the bread of life.
He who comes to me will never go hungry,
and he who believes in me will never be thirsty."
John 6:35

Often, God's best is hidden behind circumstances or relationships that appear good to us. In choosing the good, we can miss the best. During this week's study, ask God to give you a desire for His best.

DAY 1: *Receiving God's Best*

In John 6:35, the memory verse for the week, Jesus said, "He who comes to me will never go hungry." True satisfaction of your basic needs in life can only come from choosing God's source—Jesus Christ. When you are living in Him, you are experiencing the very best life God has to offer.

How appropriate that Jesus, our Bread of life, was born in Bethlehem. In Hebrew "Bethlehem" means "house of bread." When Jesus said He was the "bread of life," He declared that He is the very best spiritual nourishment you could have.

According to 2 Corinthians 5:17, you are a new creation in Christ. List ways that God has replaced the old way of life with the new.

Old	New

Does this list make you want to praise the Lord for His goodness to you? Perhaps you still have places of emptiness or hunger. The prayer of First Place is that through this program, God may fill those places. Your First Place group will also nourish you as you share and grow from their experiences.

If this is your first session with First Place, you may not be familiar with a prayer journal. It is a book with blank pages for you to fill with prayer and praise. Daily writing your prayers and requests gives you an opportunity to look back and see how God is at work in your life.

Another use for the prayer journal is to record your memory verse every day. By writing it at the top of the page every day, you will strengthen your ability to memorize the verse.

➥ What is the promise in Ezekiel 34:26?

➥ As a Christian, God gives you blessings in your life. Write some of the blessings He has given you.

Each day this week in your prayer journal write down five good things God has given you or done for you and give Him thanks. You will never run out of blessings. When you thank God for all the satisfying things He gives you, He will show you other ways He wants to satisfy your hunger through His great provision.

 Thank You, Father God, for giving me new life as a new creation in You.

Heavenly Father, show me the ways You want to satisfy my hunger through Your great provisions for my life.

DAY 2: Experiencing Drought

During the next 10 weeks, you will be studying the book of Ruth in the Old Testament. Perhaps you are familiar with this wonderful story. If not, you will grow to admire these real-life models of faithfulness.

➤ After reading Ruth 1:1-2, list the members of Elimelech's family.

Do you know what your name means? Studying biblical names often will give clues to the character and personality of the bearer. "Elimelech" means "(my) God is King." A good king provides for his people. Is it possible Elimelech lost confidence in his true King? Did he feel God was no longer able to provide because of the drought?

Elimelech left Bethlehem, the "house of bread," although others in his tribe chose to stay. He went to Moab, a pagan land. We do not know Elimelech's motives, but he never made it back home—as you will read in Ruth.

➤ According to Ruth 1:3-5, what happened to Elimelech and his sons?

Elimelech experienced a physical drought that took him to the land where he died. Many parts of our country today experience drought such as that in Bethlehem. Even more damaging is the spiritual drought that may come even when you know you are doing the things God wants you to do. Physical drought dries up the land; spiritual drought dries up the soul.

Check the box by any of the following signs of spiritual drought that you have experienced:

☐ Losing the desire to pray

☐ Having no desire to worship

☐ Feeling that the Bible doesn't speak to you anymore

☐ Avoiding Christian fellowship

Spiritually, many droughts occur because people leave home—the basic foundation of their faith. Perhaps you have stopped reading the Word or praying daily. You might have stopped going to group meetings or worship. You will often fail God's greatest tests when you are spiritually depleted. However, if you stay faithful to the basics, joy and peace will return.

➤ In 1 Corinthians 15:58, what does Paul have to say about being steadfast in God's work?

➤ Have you remained steadfast and unmovable in the work of the Lord?

☐ Yes   ☐ No   ☐ As best I can with God's help

➤ Have you experienced His love and approval for having passed a test of faith?

☐ Yes   ☐ No

Be strong in the Lord and of good courage. Return "home." Remain faithful and you will reap blessings, just as we will see that Naomi did when she returned to where she belonged after losing her husband and sons.

Lord, give me the strength and will to remain steadfast and true to Your calling for me.

Heavenly Father, prepare me for the blessings that will come to me when I remain faithful.

DAY 3: *Dwelling in Unpleasant Places*

In Ruth 1:2, you meet Naomi. Her name means "pleasant." The first thing we learn about her is that her husband moved her and their sons away to a strange place not well liked by the Israelites.

Have you ever been moved to a place that was unpleasant? Perhaps your unpleasant place was emotional or spiritual, not physical. Did you remain pleasant in the unpleasant place in your life? Did your attitudes and actions remain Christlike?

➤ In Philippians 4:11-12, what word did Paul use to describe his attitude in whatever circumstances he found himself?

➤ Name at least one circumstance during which your faith allowed you to be content, even though you were in an unpleasant situation.

➤ In 1 Thessalonians 5:18, what three-letter word did Paul use to describe circumstances for which you are to give thanks?

Is there a circumstance in your life now to which you really have not applied this principle? Do you find it difficult to respond in a pleasant way? Are you resisting and resenting the difficulty? Faith tells you that you are to rejoice in all things because God is at work, even in your difficulties.

➤ Briefly describe a time when God brought you through a difficult situation and your faith proved to be the strength you needed.

Be willing to share your experience with others who are facing difficult times. Your encouragement may be just what is needed to help them through the situation. Remember, God is always at work, even in the most unpleasant places of your life.

 Thank You, Heavenly Father, for always being at work in my life in any and every situation.

Lord, help me to be content in whatever circumstance I find myself as I rely completely on You.

DAY 4: *Keeping Commitments—Receiving Blessings*

➤ Name those who died in Ruth 1:3-4.

Naomi wanted to go back to Bethlehem, for she had heard about the Lord's blessings. She encouraged her two Moabite daughters-in-law to return to their families in Moab and start new lives while she returned to Bethlehem in Judah.

After much weeping and agony, Orpah kissed her mother-in-law good-bye and returned to her family in Moab. This decision was a perfectly normal course of action. However, Ruth took the harder path and chose to abide by her commitment to her mother-in-law.

When you examine your own level of commitment to God, do you tend to react more like Orpah or Ruth? Do you waver when difficulties come? When commitment and sacrifice are required, do you shed tears of sorrow and yet turn back?

When you joined First Place, you vowed to follow nine commitments that would bring you closer to better physical, mental, spiritual and emotional health. You may have made commitments in other areas of your life, including marriage or a commitment to a ministry. Whatever the commitment, times will arise that make keeping those commitments difficult.

➤ The following are commitments you may have made in the past. Check the ones that you have, for the most part, been able to keep.

- ☐ Daily quiet time
- ☐ First Place weekly group meetings
- ☐ Lifestyle witnessing
- ☐ Consistent exercise program
- ☐ Serving in the church
- ☐ Proper eating of balanced meals
- ☐ Prayer for fellow class members
- ☐ Encouragement of class members

Sometimes circumstances come into your life that make keeping your commitments difficult. Stress, family responsibilities, job requirements and emergencies come along to take up your time and intrude on your commitments. Although you are always encouraged to keep the nine commitments of First Place, there may be times when this is difficult. Never feel you have failed the program if you can't keep all the commitments every day, every week. Seek God's help and He will guide you every step of the way.

➤ According to Joshua 24:15, what commitment did Joshua make?

➤ At various points in your life, your commitment to God is tested and you have to decide anew to serve God. Describe a time when your commitment was tested and how you handled it.

Remember, Orpah never experienced Bethlehem, the "house of bread." She lived and died in Moab. God's biggest blessings often require the biggest commitment.

Heavenly Father, show me any areas in my life where You desire for me to have a stronger commitment to You.

Lord God, I pray that You will give me the strength and desire to keep the commitments I made to the First Place program.

DAY 5: *Becoming Beautiful in God's Eyes*

Although one of Naomi's daughters-in-law left her, the other daughter-in-law remained faithful. She is the person for whom the Bible book is named—Ruth. "Ruth" means "sightly." Was Ruth a beautiful woman? We have no way of knowing. However, we do know she represents a person with a beautiful commitment in the eyes of the Lord. It might be said that such a person has a beautiful heart.

➤ Describe a committed heart in your own words, based on 1 Kings 8:61.

➤ On a scale of 1 to 10, with 10 as totally committed, how committed is your own heart? Circle your answer.

1   2   3   4   5   6   7   8   9   1   0

God looks for Christians with committed hearts, so He can display His power through them. One of the greatest testimonies of God's power occurs when you make a firm commitment to better physical health and fitness. These changes are visually evident and are difficult to make without the strength and help of the Lord. When you are healthier, the question will always arise, How did you do it? What a perfect opportunity for you to share about God's power. Real beauty is not just a pleasing physical presence, but it is also a heart that glorifies God.

➤ Think of people you know. Write the names of those whose commitment and love of the Lord make them beautiful.

A committed heart in service to Him is beautiful. What could be more beautiful to God than one of His children giving Him glory continuously by becoming and staying fit and healthy? Do you have a desire for others around you to see God's power through you? They can see Him clearly if your commitment is wholehearted.

You come into contact with people every day who don't know the Lord as their personal Savior. Your life may touch theirs daily or only on an occasional basis. What is their life worth to the Lord? Is it worth your commitment of time and effort to show them how strong God is in you?

➤ List the people you know who need the Lord.

Keep the list to remind you that your witness to them will be greatly increased as you succeed in your commitments to First Place.

Heavenly Father, give me the desire and determination I need to make a commitment to better health and fitness through the First Place program.

Dear Lord, inspire me to become a beautiful person in Your eyes with a heart and mind fully focused on You. Let others see Your love through me.

DAY 6: *Reflections*

As you complete this first week of the study, our desire is for you to see the importance of ministry to the whole person, not just your physical health. Whatever the reason for your joining the program, we pray that you will grow in all areas of your life.

Our main emphasis during these days of reflection will be on memorizing and praying God's Word. The Bible is full of beautiful passages of Scripture that fulfill every need in your life. Memorizing those Scriptures gives you a weapon of great power to conquer any strongholds that may attempt to crowd out the Holy Spirit at work in your life. A stronghold is defined in 2 Corinthians 10:5 as "arguments and every pretension that sets itself up against the knowledge of God."

In *Praying God's Word*, Beth Moore addresses the various strongholds that can weaken a person and make him or her a less effective witness to the power of God.[1] The Bible tells you to "take captive every thought to make it obedient to Christ" (2 Corinthians 10:5). Verse 4 tells us that the weapons we possess "have divine power to demolish strongholds."

You already know the power of prayer. Think of the combined power of the Word of God and prayer. As modeled in Beth's book, combining the Word of God and prayer results in a mighty arsenal that will send Satan fleeing in fear. He can't hold on when such power is exhibited in your life. No matter what your stronghold may be, God's power and grace will help you overcome it through the Holy Spirit. Strongholds don't come on suddenly overnight. It takes months and even years to build up and support a stronghold, and it may take months and years to demolish it, or God may choose to destroy it completely overnight or in a few days.

The point is not to be discouraged. Continue to hide God's Word in your heart and to pray for His mighty power to enable you to be a conqueror.

Strengthen your battle with Scripture memory. Use your prayer journal or any other means you desire to write down verses with special meaning to you. Review them every day along with your memory verse of the week. Use them in your prayers and in your conversations and correspondence with others. When you send an encouraging word or call a fellow class member, use the week's verse to give strength to both of you.

O Lord, be my rock of refuge, to which I can always go; give the command to save me, for You are my rock and my fortress (see Psalm 71:3).[2]

In my anguish I cry to You, Lord. Answer me by setting me free! You, the Lord, are with me; I will not be afraid. The Lord is with me; He is my helper. I will look in triumph on my enemy (see Psalm 118:5-7).[3]

Dear Lord, please lead me not into temptation, but deliver me from the evil one (see Matthew 6:13).[4]

DAY 7: *Reflections*

Your first response to being asked to memorize Scripture might be "But I can't memorize that much Scripture!" You're not alone. Many who came before you said the same thing. We give you many aids and methods to help you memorize. Make your first goal the memory verse for the week. Write it down and listen to the Scripture Memory Verses CD. Take *Walking in the Word* with you wherever you go. Each time you have a moment, read your memory verse. Listen to your CD while driving. Remember to use the verse when you communicate with others and include it in your written messages.

Using the memory verse as a basis for a prayer is another way to help implant the words in your heart and mind. While you are praying, use several Scriptures that come to mind as you think of various needs in your life and the lives of others. In the beginning, you may not be able to quote the verse word for word; but with repetition, the words will come.

One important aspect of memorizing God's Word is to make it your Scripture and have it so ingrained in your heart that you automatically turn to those verses in times of stress, rather than fretting and worrying about situations. No situation is so difficult that God and prayer cannot help. He may not undo the entire incident, but He will definitely give you peace about what is happening. Some things you can alter with a change in your behavior or attitude; others cannot be changed by human means. If change is entirely out of your control, you can put it completely in God's control.

An example of this happened to an older woman who was diagnosed with breast cancer. She knew she could do nothing to physically alter the diagnosis, but she knew God could alter it. She prayed using the words of Matthew 21:22. Surgeons removed the cancer and discovered no further occurrence. No lymph nodes were involved and the doctor decided against radiation or chemotherapy. The cancer was gone when the tumors were removed. The surgeon expressed surprise; the woman expressed her thanks to God.

Whether you are a visual, auditory or hands-on learner, you can find a method of memorizing Scripture that will best suit you. The important thing is the desire to know God's Word and memorize it. When the sincere desire is there, the Holy Spirit will work through you.

The following are Bible verses that meet special needs. The need is listed and then the prayer using an appropriate Scripture passage. The last example is this week's verse as a prayer.

Patience

Heavenly Father, I pray that I not become lazy. Help me to imitate those who through faith and patience inherit what has been promised (see Hebrews 6:12).

Emotional Baggage

Holy Lord, help me to cast my cares on You, for You will sustain me; You will never permit the righteous to fall (see Psalm 55:22).

Burnout

O Father, grant me the rest You promised to all those weary and heavily burdened who come to You (see Matthew 11:28).

Father God, You have promised never to leave me nor forsake me. Help me to feel Your presence today (see Hebrews 13:5b).

Bitterness

Holy God, help me get rid of all bitterness, rage, anger, brawling and slander, along with every form of malice. Keep my heart and mind steadfastly on You (see Ephesians 4:31).

Memory Verse

Oh, Father, You have said You are the bread of life; and those who come to You will never go hungry and those who believe in You will never be thirsty. Fill my hunger and thirst with Your Word (see John 6:35).

Notes
1. Beth Moore, *Praying God's Word* (Nashville, TN: Broadman and Holman, 2000).
2. Ibid., p. 322.
3. Ibid., p. 324.
4. Ibid., p. 326.

GROUP PRAYER REQUESTS   TODAY'S DATE:_____

NAME	REQUEST	RESULTS

COMMITTED TO RETURNING

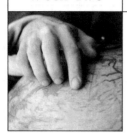

MEMORY VERSE
*"Ever since the time of your forefathers you have
turned away from my decrees and have not kept them.
Return to me, and I will return to you,"*
says the LORD Almighty.
Malachi 3:7

The people of God often find themselves in a foreign land—or a place away from God—just as Naomi did after the death of her husband and sons. Just as the desire to return to the place of God's blessings will draw us back to Him, in this week's study we will discover the five steps necessary for returning to the blessings of the Lord.

DAY 1: *Go Where He Goes*

The first chapter of Ruth contains verses familiar to many wedding participants.

➤ Read Ruth 1:15-18. Why do you think verses 16 and 17 are often read at wedding ceremonies?

This passage is one of the most beautiful expressions of commitment in the Bible and it illustrates the five steps of returning to the will of God. The first step is found in the statement "Where you go I will go." Be ready to go when the Lord tells you to go. Often the will of the Lord for your life takes a new direction, and you are not ready or willing to make the change. This change can be physical, geographical, philosophical or relational. You must not let the Lord leave without you!

➤ Describe a time when the Lord had a change for the plans you had made.

➤ Which type of change would you say it was?

☐ A place
☐ A belief
☐ A job
☐ A relationship
☐ A lifestyle issue
☐ Other _____

In order for Ruth to reach the place of blessing, she had to go where Naomi went. She had to trust Naomi to know the way. She could not just go part of the way to receive the blessing. Like Ruth, you must be willing to follow where the Lord takes you and to not give up following. Trust His tender mercies and He will be your guide.

➤ In John 12:26, what does Jesus tell you to do, and what is the reward?

➤ In what ways or areas have you resisted change or neglected to follow His will?

Let go and give God full reign in your life. Make the commitment in your own life to go where He goes. Follow Jesus Christ with all your heart.

Examine my heart, O God. Show me Your way and lead me in the right path.

Lord, give me a willing heart to make a commitment to You and to follow You in all areas of my life.

DAY 2: *Stop When He Stops*

In addition to being willing to go where God goes, you must be willing to stop when He stops. You can be just as much out of the Lord's will if you move ahead of Him as when you lag behind Him. This second step to returning to God's blessings occurs in Ruth's request to Naomi.

➳ In Ruth 1:16, what two things does Ruth tell Naomi not to ask again?

   1.

   2.

Ruth knew she would be separated from Naomi if she did either of these things. Ruth said, "Where you stay I will stay." Moving ahead of God separates you from His close fellowship.

➳ Describe a time when you got in a hurry and ran ahead of God.

➳ What were the results of moving ahead of God's plan?

➳ What does the psalmist say about waiting on the Lord in Psalm 27:14?

Waiting on the Lord and His timing does take courage and heart. In First Place, you can move ahead of God if you become impatient with your progress. You may be tempted to try to lose weight by false methods such as using diet pills or other "no pain" methods because you want to reach your goal *now*. Part of maturing in Christ is learning to take small steps of faith that produce long-term results.

➤ What does John 10:25-30 say about the blessings of being one of His sheep?

➤ How does this make you feel?

Dear Lord, show me the areas where I need to listen for Your voice, so I will follow You and not try to lead or get ahead.

Heavenly Father, help me to be still and wait patiently on Your timing for the things You have planned for me.

DAY 3: *Love Those He Loves*

The third step in returning to God's blessings is found in the phrase "Your people will be my people," in Ruth 1:16. Ruth was willing to forsake her family and friends in Moab to become part of Naomi's family in Bethlehem. In a similar fashion, you cannot be part of the Lord's family if you hang on to worldly relationships.

➤ What does 1 John 4:20 call a person who says he loves God but hates his Christian brother?

Have you ever heard Christians say they do not attend church because they don't like other Christians? When you really love someone, you care about the person regardless of his or her flaws. If you really love the Lord, you will love the Church, which is made up of His people.

➤ Check the following that best describes your love for the people of your church.

□ I love everyone at my church.

□ I don't like some people at my church.

□ I love most of them, but I don't know many of the people at my church.

□ I don't feel love for them because I'm not very active in my church.

➤ List some ways church members show their Christlike love for each other.

Sometimes church members may think they have to know people to really love them. Ruth didn't know Naomi's family in Bethlehem, but she loved them because she loved Naomi. The same is true for us when we love the Lord Jesus. You should not stay away from His church because you don't like a certain person or people. He loves them and you love Him. You can accept other believers and trust Him to work in their lives as well as your own.

➤ Considering Ephesians 1:6-8, what does it mean to you to feel accepted by God?

In your prayer journal make a list of people you may not have accepted for one reason or another. Ask God to help you accept them because He loves them.

Heavenly Father, thank You for loving me and giving Your Son, Jesus Christ, to die for me. Help me to love others as You have loved me.

Lord, give me opportunities in my church family to demonstrate the love You commanded us to have for one another.

DAY 4: *Worship the One True God*

The next step in returning to the center of God's blessing involves your worship of Him. In Ruth's confession of faithfulness in 1:16 she tells Naomi, "Your God [will be] my God." Ruth was from a pagan society. She only knew of God because of the witness of her new family. She desired to worship the one true God.

Worship of the Lord is a key to your relationship with Him. The more you worship Him, the more you will love Him. Certainly, especially after a spiritual drought, you need to truly worship Him. In John 4:21-24, Jesus talks with a woman at a well about worship requirements.

➤ What are the two requirements for true worship (v. 24)?

These two words reveal how Jesus worshiped His heavenly Father. The Spirit brings life to an otherwise dead ritual, or performance. The Spirit enables you to have true communion with God. To worship in truth means you worship the true God.

➤ How did Jesus describe Himself in John 14:6?

➤ What does Romans 10:9-13 tell us about being saved?

➤ Have you ever honestly and sincerely called on the name of the Lord and asked Him to become your Savior?

☐ Yes ☐ No

➤ If your answer is yes, write the time and place when this wonderful life-changing experience happened to you.

If your answer is no, will you ask Christ to become your Lord and Savior based on the promise He made in Romans 10:13? Simply pray the following prayer from the depths of your own heart right now:

Heavenly Father, forgive me for all of my sins. Jesus, please come into my heart and save me through Your sacrificial death on the cross. Thank You for saving me, Lord Jesus. I take You as the Lord of my life. In Jesus' name I pray. Amen.

If you sincerely prayed and asked Christ to save you, He did. You are now a Christian and will go to heaven when you die. Write today's date in the margin, so you will have a permanent record of your salvation experience. Be sure to tell your First Place leader, your pastor or another Christian about your decision.

Heavenly Father, thank You for the Holy Spirit now living in me.

Lord Jesus, I come to worship You in spirit and in truth for You are the way, the truth and the life.

DAY 5: Stay as Long as He Stays

Have you ever visited a scenic or famous place only to realize you will probably never see it again? When Ruth looked back at Moab, she knew she was seeing it for the last time.

➤ According to Ruth 1:17, how long was Ruth willing to live in Bethlehem and keep her commitment to Naomi?

☐ Until she married
☐ Until Naomi died
☐ Until she died

Ruth was willing to live in Bethlehem the rest of her life. In fact, she planned to be buried there.

The fifth and last step to returning to God's blessing after a time of dryness represents a giant commitment. You realize you must never go back to your Moab again. In fact you must die to Moab—your old way of life—altogether. Close the door to your old way of life and become a new creature because of your salvation and commitment to the Lord. Even if you temporarily look back, God is faithful to provide a way back to your new lifestyle.

➤ In what ways did your lifestyle change when you became a Christian?

➤ What things do you do as a Christian that you didn't (or wouldn't) do as a non-Christian?

➤ In what ways has your lifestyle changed since you began First Place?

➤ How long are you committed to this change?

➣ According to Colossians 3:1-5, where are we to set our hearts and minds?

➣ What happened to your life when you became a Christian?

➣ What must we put to death?

Just as Ruth committed to following Naomi and staying with her all her life, your Christian commitment is for a lifetime. The significant difference is that your commitment to Jesus goes beyond earthly life to eternal life with Him. Are you setting your mind and life on godly things? God will help you make the commitment to let your life be a reflection of Him in your heart and mind.

Heavenly Father, help me to live out my commitment to You on a daily basis by keeping my mind steadfast on You for the rest of my life.

Lord God, may my life always be a reflection of You, so others may see Your love and mercy at work in me.

DAY 6: *Reflections*

This week's lesson focuses on the lifetime commitment of Ruth and your lifetime commitment to Jesus Christ. Once you become a Christian, you need to change your lifestyle and live for Him every day. When you slip and fall into temptation or when something in your life other than the Holy Spirit wants to take over, God is there to keep you on track or to bring you back to His way.

The same principle is true with your First Place commitment. Once you change your lifestyle to include good eating habits, exercise, Bible study, prayer and memorizing Scripture, you follow it for a lifetime. Whenever you allow bad habits to get in the way and you fall back into old patterns, the Holy Spirit will help you break free and return to a healthier way of life.

If you look at First Place as a lifetime commitment rather than a diet-and-lose-weight-until-I-reach-my-goal program, you will find greater satisfaction and success in what you are doing, and your lifestyle will let others see what God can do.

In addition to changing your lifestyle to healthy eating and good habits, you are developing a lifestyle that leads to a closer, more intimate relationship with God. If prayer and Bible study have not been a part of your daily routine, the First Place commitments will help you to do so. Memorizing Scripture will become easier for you as you read His Word, study it and pray on a regular basis. Are you in this lifestyle for the long haul or just to reach some short-term goal? Return to Him and He promises to bless you.

The following Scripture prayers speak to your dedication and perseverance to make First Place your new lifestyle:

For I know that my old self was crucified with You, Christ, so that this body of sin might be done away with, that I should no longer be a slave to sin—because anyone who has died has been freed from sin (see Romans 6:6-7).[1]

You, Lord, will rescue me from every evil attack and will bring me safely to Your heavenly kingdom. To You be glory for ever and ever (see 2 Timothy 4:18).[2]

I am Your dear child, and I am from You, God, and have overcome the influences of the evil kingdom, because the One who is in me is greater than the one who is in the world (see 1 John 4:4).[3]

DAY 7: *Reflections*

Once you commit to a lifestyle change for life, you need tools to help you keep your commitment. These tools are also the weapons with which you battle Satan. He wants you to slip and fall away from your commitments, but you have all you need to defeat his schemes.

Memorizing Scripture and quoting verses as you pray bring fear to Satan and he has to flee from you in defeat. Once you are "dead to sin" (Romans 6:11), your desire to please God and nourish the Holy Spirit will give you power to memorize the Bible verses you select as your weapons in your spiritual battle against Satan. Be assured that Satan will not leave you alone. Indeed, he works even harder once your life is committed to Christ.

Satan will help you come up with all kinds of excuses to prevent you from fulfilling your commitments to the First Place program. Your greatest defense is a strong offense, and that offense is strengthened by Scripture and prayer. Through prayer and Bible study, you take captive all your thoughts and make them obedient to Christ. Your reward is a closer intimacy with God. In *Praying God's Word*, Beth Moore writes, "I finally learned that the way to make our exalted, overpowering thoughts bow down in obedience to Jesus Christ is to choose to think His thoughts about the matter rather than my own or those influenced by the enemy."[4] This goes along with the popular saying "What would Jesus do?"

Put on the whole armor of God with the sword of the Spirit foremost and go into battle with confidence. God is on your side and will give you the victory.

Heavenly Father, thank You for the weapons of warfare which are not of this world but have divine power to demolish strongholds (see 2 Corinthians 10:4).

Lord God, it is for freedom that Christ has set me free. Help me to stand firm, and do not let me be burdened again by a yoke of slavery (see Galatians 5:1).

Dear Lord, let me not become weary in doing good, for I know that at the proper time I will reap a harvest if I do not give up (see Galatians 6:9).

Notes
1. Beth Moore, *Praying God's Word* (Nashville, TN: Broadman and Holman, 2000), p. 154.
2. Ibid., p. 157.
3. Ibid.
4. Ibid., p. 7.

GROUP PRAYER REQUESTS   TODAY'S DATE:_____

NAME	REQUEST	RESULTS

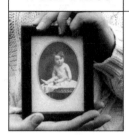

MEMORY VERSE

Give thanks in all circumstances,
for this is God's will for you in Christ Jesus.
1 Thessalonians 5:18

How do you think the residents of Bethlehem reacted to Naomi's return? What did they think of her Moabite daughter-in-law? Naomi had definitely changed since she left home many years before.

In this week's Bible study, you will reflect on how you have changed over the years and whether those changes have been mostly positive or mostly negative.

DAY 1: *Experiencing a Joyous Welcome*

Have you ever returned home after being gone for an extended period of time? Didn't you feel relief at finally being back in your own surroundings? Have you ever attended a reunion either with family or old friends? Was there a buzz of excitement at seeing family and friends not seen for a long time? Put yourself in Naomi's position. Imagine what she must have been thinking and feeling as she saw Bethlehem on the horizon.

➤ According to Ruth 1:19, what was the response of the city when they saw Naomi?

The word "stirred" implies that a literal uproar broke out in the whole city when Ruth and Naomi arrived. It must have been reassuring to Naomi that the whole town remembered her.

If you have faced or are facing a Moab experience—a time of being uprooted physically, emotionally or spiritually—the Lord gives a joyous welcome when you return to Him. You may think God will be angry with you, but Scripture does not characterize God this way. Luke 15:11-32 relates the familiar story of the prodigal son.

➤ In verse 20, what was the father's reaction to seeing his son coming home?

➤ What was the son's reply in verse 21?

God wants his family to be united. Every time a forgiven child strays and then returns, great rejoicing takes place.

➤ Read Hebrews 10:25. Why does the Lord want us to meet together as believers?

Think of a time when you had a spiritual drought, or Moab experience, and distanced yourself from your fellow Christians or your First Place group. Were you hesitant to return to the group because you expected rejection? Did you get a warm welcome home, rather than a rejection?

➤ Describe the experience you had.

If Satan can keep you separated from other believers, your recovery is less likely. To keep you from returning to them and fellowshiping with the Lord, he will lie, saying you have shamed your friends and family. You will always find a warm welcome, rather than rejection, when you come humbly and gratefully back to Jesus.

Perhaps there is an individual or group to whom you need to return and reestablish fellowship. Pray about the situation and return to them and know the joy of restoration.

 Heavenly Father, thank You for loving me and welcoming me back when I stray from Your family.

Father God, instill in me a forgiving heart and help me to welcome back with open arms and a warm heart any who have strayed and now return.

DAY 2: *Rekindling Joy*

Naomi's return to Bethlehem certainly did not go unnoticed! The women exclaimed, "Is this Naomi?" (see Ruth 1:19). They were asking if this was the woman named "pleasant." Were they expecting the same pleasant woman who had left Bethlehem years earlier?

➤ What was Naomi's response in Ruth 1:20-21 to the people of Bethlehem when they called her name?

➤ The Hebrew word *Mara* means "bitter." Why would Naomi want to be called bitter instead of pleasant?

The people of the town acted as if she were still the same pleasant Naomi. Have any of life's circumstances produced bitterness in you? Review the memory verse for this week.

≫ Has there been a time in your life when you felt you had no joy because of your circumstances? Briefly describe the experience.

≫ According to Psalm 51:12, what is the one joy the Lord is always willing to restore?

≫ According to Psalm 51:10, what else will God give you?

No matter how far away you may go or what bitterness and/or sadness you may face, God loves you and is willing to restore your joy and give you a clean heart and a steadfast spirit.

Lord, if there be any qualities I have left behind over the years, help me to reclaim them for Your glory.

Father, I pray for a clean heart and steadfast spirit so that I may be a more effective witness of Your great love and mercy.

DAY 3: *Acknowledging Bitterness*

Naomi was no longer pleasant but bitter. Staying away from godly people has the potential to change your disposition. The longer you distance yourself from His will, the more bitterness can grow. If you remain in a spiritual drought long enough, it will even begin to affect your family and others around you.

≫ According to Hebrews 12:14-15, what happens when bitterness invades our lives?

✎ What characteristics can help you avoid bitterness?

✎ Read Ephesians 4:30-32. How would bitterness affect the Holy Spirit's work in your life?

✎ What did Paul tell you to do instead of being bitter?

✎ Describe your spiritual fullness or emptiness at this time by checking one of the following statements:

☐ I am as close to the Lord as I have ever been.
☐ I am almost as close as ever.
☐ I am not as close as I have been.
☐ I am as far from the Lord as I have ever been since salvation.

✎ Is there any bitterness or unresolved hurt in your life? Describe it.

✎ How could you get rid of bitterness or hurt in your life?

Just as we would rid ourselves of any sin by confession, we can confess bitterness and ask God to remove it from our lives.

Dear Lord, help me to get beyond any hurt or bitterness in my life and return me to the joy that only You can give.

Heavenly Father, grant me wisdom to know how to guard against the bitter root that can grow up to cause trouble and hurt others.

DAY 4: *Seeing Yourself Through God's Eyes*

Naomi wanted to be called Mara. She no longer looked at herself through God's eyes but through the eyes of pain. Bitterness will cause you to look at yourself through the eyes of hurt and not through the eyes of the Lord.

➺ What did Paul say about suffering in Romans 8:18?

In this verse Paul was not bitter because of his suffering. He knew his suffering was not a result of disobedience but because he was obedient. Rather than exercising his right to a pity party or wanting to run away from pain, he looked at himself through the eyes of the Lord, rather than the eyes of hurt. He saw that his suffering could glorify the Lord.

➺ List one or more difficulties in your life from which the Lord received glory.

➺ Are you able to look back with a thankful heart at these difficulties? Why?

➺ Do you believe God allowed these events to come into your life to help you and not hurt you? Why?

➤ Are you more like Him today because of your experience? Explain.

Once when Michelangelo was asked how he could make a beautifully sculptured horse out of an ugly chunk of dirty marble, he simply replied, "I take a hammer and chisel and I knock off everything that doesn't look like a horse." Sometimes the Lord uses difficulties to knock off everything from our lives that doesn't look like Him. He sees a beautiful creation hidden under our hard exterior.

The Lord will help you to look past your pain and see His purpose in your hardship.

Heavenly Father, help me to see my life through Your eyes and know that You only want what is good for me.

Thank You, Lord, for those things You bring my way to make me more like Christ.

DAY 5: *Yielding to God's Helping Hand*

Many times when bitterness comes into a person's life, he or she will try to blame it on someone else much as Adam blamed Eve and Eve blamed the serpent for their sin in Genesis. Naomi blamed someone for the bitterness that came into her life. Read Ruth 1:20-21.

➤ Verse 20: "The Almighty has made my life very_____."

➤ Verse 21: "The Almighty has brought _____
upon me."

Naomi believed that the Lord was against her because of the deaths of her husband and sons. Grief and loss may lead some to feel completely abandoned by the heavenly Father. Some even blame God for the way they look or the way they're made. Be assured, God made you the way you are to bless you. Through the disciplines of the nine commitments of First Place, you can experience His love. Discipline is guidance, not punishment. Discipline is love.

Parents discipline children because they love them, not because they want to harm them. God's discipline is out of love, not the lack of it. When you look at God's discipline as hurtful, you mistake His helping, healing hand for a hurtful, harmful one.

➤ What does Hebrews 12:5-7 say to you about God's discipline?

➤ Can you remember a time in your own life when your earthly parents' correction seemed to be hurting you, when actually they were helping you?

A First Place member recalled this incident from his childhood:

I was playing near a large bluff that my father had told me to stay away from. One day, while playing with a friend, I decided to jump from the upper level to the lower level. I didn't realize how difficult it would be for a chubby boy like me to climb back up. After what seemed like hours, I gave up and asked my friend to get my father. I knew I was in big trouble. My father came and didn't say a word to me. He just reached with his large hand and grabbed my wrist and began to pull me up the cliff to safety. When I got to the top, he hugged me and asked if I was OK. He never mentioned it again, and I never played near that cliff again. I had mistaken my father's helping hand for his hurting hand.

➤ What is the message of Proverbs 3:11-12 for your life?

⋙ In Hebrews 12:10, God gives you another reason for His discipline. What is it?

If God loves you so much that He wants you to share in His Holiness, then His discipline is to be looked upon as guidance toward Him and the blessings He can bestow.

⋙ Considering 1 Thessalonians 5:16-18, what are you to do when God's discipline comes?

Heavenly Father, help me to be content and give thanks for Your helping hand when You show Your love through discipline.

Dear God, take away any bitterness I may have as a result of any hurt I may feel because I mistook Your helping hand for a harmful one.

DAY 6: *Reflections*

This week you have learned about the discipline of God and how much He loves you. So many times you make choices and decisions in life that are not in God's will. These decisions and choices may bring difficulties into your life. God lovingly shows you the way back, although you may wonder, *Why is He allowing these things to happen to me?*

Today it seems everyone is trying to shift the blame for his or her actions on someone else. So many want to blame a deprived childhood, abusive parents, poverty and anything else they can think of for the condition they are in. They simply do not want to take responsibility for their actions.

As a Christian, every decision you make, every choice you make, should be based on what you learn from reading God's Word and seeking His will for your life. When wrong decisions or choices are made, you may suffer consequences that hurt. When this happens, remember your loving heavenly Father will comfort and see you through the problem.

Whether you are making a decision or suffering through the consequences of a poor decision, God's Word gives you the guidance you need. Scripture memorization plays an important role in how you make a decision or how you respond to consequences.

In times of trouble or indecision, trust God's Word. Having Scripture written on your heart gives you an instant resource, and you don't have to wait until you can look it up in the Bible. You now have at least three memory verses. If you have not memorized them yet, make a special effort over the next few days to write those words in your heart and mind. Use the *Walking in the Word* book and your CDs as aids. Write the verses on cards or paper. Use whatever method is best for you, but seal them in your heart and mind.

The following sentence prayers are based on Scripture concerning the discipline of God as a loving Father:

Heavenly Father, help me to understand Your discipline and not despise it or resent Your rebuke, because I know that You discipline those You love as a father disciplines a son he loves (see Proverbs 3:11-12).

Lord God, because You rebuke and discipline those You love, help me to be earnest and repent of my sin (see Revelation 3:19).

Gracious Lord, help me remember that no discipline seems pleasant at the time, but it will produce a harvest of righteousness and peace (see Hebrews 12:11).

DAY 7: *Reflections*

No matter in what situation you may find yourself, you will find a verse in God's Word to get you through. When your heart is full of love and thanksgiving, God's Word will give you the words of thanks you need to praise Him. When you stray away from your commitment to Him, the Scriptures will guide you back to His loving grace.

What better reasons could you have for memorizing God's Word? If you're still having problems with memorizing, enlist the help of a friend who will listen to you repeat the verse until you can do it easily. Your friend can provide encouragement to you as you say the words. In turn, you can encourage your friend as he or she memorizes.

Memorizing Scripture brings to your mind a truth you need in time of difficulty, when temptation comes or when seeking guidance for your life. When you have an opportunity to witness, God's Word will provide the means to impart the truth. Memorized verses become a powerful aid when you are seeking to console or give encouragement to a friend. With God's truths in your heart and mind, you have the resource for any and every situation.

Father God, I don't want to grieve You. Remove from me all bitterness, rage, anger, brawling and slander along with every form of malice (see Ephesians 4:30-31).

Heavenly Father, though You have made me see troubles, many and bitter, You will restore my life again; from the depths of the earth You will bring me up (see Psalm 71:20).

Lord, do not let me sin in my anger. Do not let the sun go down while I am still angry. Help me to resolve anger, so the devil does not get a foothold (see Ephesians 4:26-27).

Dear Lord, help me to give thanks in all circumstances for this is God's will for me in Christ Jesus (see 1 Thessalonians 5:18).

GROUP PRAYER REQUESTS TODAY'S DATE:_____

NAME	REQUEST	RESULTS

BEGINNING A LOVE RELATIONSHIP

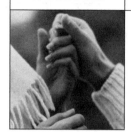

MEMORY VERSE

While we wait for the blessed hope—the glorious appearing of our great God and Savior, Jesus Christ, who gave himself for us to redeem us from all wickedness and to purify for himself a people that are his very own, eager to do what is good.
Titus 2:13-14

This week's study shifts focus from Naomi to Ruth, a Gentile who had never been to Bethlehem. As you follow her adjustments, look for ways Ruth's experience parallels your own as you once began, and now continue, a love relationship with God and His people.

DAY 1: *A Divine Appointment*

Remember that Bethlehem in Judah—the "house of bread"—symbolizes God's very best for you. Christ is the Bread of Life and worthy of all our praise. In chapter 1 of the book of Ruth, Naomi returned to God's best after living away from Him. In chapter 2, as Ruth comes to Bethlehem for the first time, her life might remind you of your first encounters with God. With God you can always have a new beginning.

➽ According to Ruth 2:1-3, what was Boaz's relationship to Naomi?

➽ What was his position in the community?

Ruth went out to find food in the barley fields of the area. The poor and hungry were allowed to pick up the grain that the harvesters dropped or left behind; this process is called gleaning.

➤ According to Ruth 2:3, how did Ruth get into the field that belonged to Boaz?

Ruth's choice may have seemed to be happenstance from an earthly viewpoint, but from God's viewpoint it was a divine appointment. Things don't just happen when God sets them into motion. Just as He had a plan for Ruth, He has a plan for you.

➤ Describe a time when you experienced a divine appointment to fulfill God's plan in your life.

➤ How might joining First Place or beginning this study be a divine appointment for you?

➤ How does Jeremiah 29:11-13 help you understand God's plan for your life?

Thank You, Heavenly Father, for caring for me and having plans for me that will prosper me and give me a hope and a future.

Thank You, Lord, for all the things that You provide. Help me to recognize divine appointments that You send my way.

DAY 2: *The Plight of an Outsider*

According to Jewish law, when a married man died without a male heir, his next of kin was obligated to marry his widow and raise his children in the name of the deceased man. If the next of kin were unable to do so, then the next male relative in line was given the responsibility. This practice allowed the land to stay in the family because land could only pass from father to son.

➤ To which woman did the law in Deuteronomy 25:5-6 apply? Circle your answer.

   Naomi   Ruth   Orpah

This practice was especially important in Bethlehem because eventually the Messiah would be born to the tribe of Judah. You must remember, however, that Ruth was a Gentile and a Moabite. Moabites were among the least welcomed by the Jewish people. This attitude was even commanded in Scripture (see Deuteronomy 23:3-6).

➤ Describe how you think Ruth must have felt those first days in Bethlehem.

Ruth was an outsider with no hope of gaining admission into the exclusive Jewish nation. Yet her story is not finished. Like Ruth, until we meet our Redeemer, Jesus Christ, we are outsiders—alone with no hope of eternal life in heaven.

Do you recall a time when you felt like an outsider? Perhaps when you went to a new school, went off to college, met your in-laws the first time, joined a new church or joined a new group where you didn't know anyone.

➤ Describe the time you felt like an outsider.

- What helped you feel included in, or a part of, the group?

- As a child of God, what does Ephesians 2:11-13 mean to you?

Put yourself in Ruth's place and think about what it might have been like to have been an outsider in the Hebrew nation.

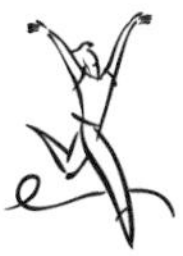

Thank You, Heavenly Father, for my salvation and for making me a member of the family of God.

Dear Lord, help me to always welcome newcomers to my church or to my group with open arms and a loving heart.

DAY 3: *The Price of Redemption*

In the Jewish society the oldest male relative was called the kinsman-redeemer. He was responsible for redeeming, or buying back, any land or possessions lost to the family. There were several ways property could leave a family's ownership.

It could be given away. It could be sold for money to live on. It could be stolen or taken by those who dishonestly took advantage of families in distress. It could be lost through illness or death.

The kinsman-redeemer had to have the wealth to pay the price of redemption. In a similar way, the Lord Jesus had to be able to pay a price to redeem us from our state of spiritual poverty.

- According to Romans 3:23-24 and 6:23, what is your condition without God?

➤ Who is the source of your redemption?

➤ What is the result of sin?

➤ In contrast, what is the gift of God?

➤ What does 2 Corinthians 5:21 tell you about God's redemption plan?

Since the wages, or debt, of sin is death and Christ knew no sin, it would also follow that He owed no debt of death. He was rich in the righteousness necessary to be our Savior. Jesus owed nothing, yet He paid a price because you, His child, could not pay the debt you owed. To be redeemed, you simply accept His payment of death on the cross.

Reflect on and write a brief testimony about your own salvation experience. If you have not accepted Christ as your Savior, speak to your leader about doing this. You can also experience the wonderful grace and love of God through Jesus' redemptive death on the cross. The Holy Spirit will come and be your comforter and guide.

 Thank You, Lord Jesus, for Your free gift of grace that I could not earn and do not deserve.

Thank You, Jesus, for loving me. Help me to live a healthy lifestyle as an offering back to You for Your great gift of eternal life.

DAY 4: A Claim for God's Blessing

When Ruth and Naomi came to Bethlehem, they struggled for even a meager existence. God had an abundant future in store for them, but they had not yet experienced His rich blessings. Do you think they even dared to hope for a better life? Does God want you to ask Him for blessings?

➦ According to John 10:10, what three things does Christ say the "thief" has come to do?

➦ What did Jesus come to do?

➦ What is your definition of having life to the full?

The thief in this passage is the devil himself. The devil wants to steal that which is yours as a member of God's family. He wants to steal your joy, peace and victory. These are the things restored to you when you are reborn into the family of God.

➦ What is the fullness Paul describes in Colossians 2:9-10?

The Lord created you to experience His very best. His joy, peace, victory and power were meant for His children to possess and enjoy. Just as the kinsman-redeemer restored his family's possessions, our Kinsman-redeemer—Christ—restores what is rightfully ours as family members and heirs of the Kingdom. You must not live beneath your privilege as a child of the King of kings.

✎ According to Romans 12:1, what is your responsibility as a Christian?

✎ How does this relate to your belonging to a First Place group?

Presenting yourself as a living sacrifice involves the mind, heart, soul and body. All must work together to be holy and pleasing to the Lord. God is not pleased when you abuse your health. Everything you do must be "holy and pleasing to God—this is your spiritual act of worship" (Romans 12:1).

Heavenly Father, help me to claim those qualities in my life that I need to make my body a living sacrifice to You.

Lord Jesus, thank You for the many blessings You bestow on me as a member of the family of God.

DAY 5: *Heirs of God's Blessings*

As you have already learned, one of the duties of the kinsman-redeemer was to raise children in his brother's name. Having an heir was essential in Jewish society. Jesus' death and resurrection allow you to become a child of God! Through the gift of eternal life, you are born again as a joint heir with Christ!

✎ According to Galatians 3:26—4:7, what does it mean to be an heir?

✎ Who was included in those who could become heirs?

How do you become a member of God's family?

Heirs might pass on blessings of their inheritance to others. When you share your salvation experience, you are spreading the gospel, or good news, of your redeemer and how He welcomed you into His family, even when you were an outsider.

What is Paul's testimony in Romans 1:16?

Name some people with whom you have shared or intend to share the plan of salvation.

The testimony of your First Place experience can be a starting point to open doors for witnessing.

If you were unable to list any names, would you be willing to ask God to bring a person into your life with whom you can share the good news?

☐ Yes   ☐ No

The New Testament contains many examples of people who were eager to share the gospel of Jesus Christ with others. One is the Samaritan woman described in John 4:7-29, while another is the disciple Andrew described in John 1:40-42.

What was the woman's testimony in John 4:7-29?

~~ What was Andrew's testimony in John 1:40-42?

If you checked yes above, then you must be ready and willing to share the good news of Christ's redemption every time God gives you the opportunity. Jesus came to redeem everyone. Your love relationship with Him begins at the point of salvation. It matures as you join Him in His work in the world. Review this week's memory verse. If you ask God, He will reveal ways for you to demonstrate your eagerness to do good as you go about your responsibilities.

 Heavenly Father, give me a boldness to go out and share the message of salvation with those who don't know You.

DAY 6: *Reflections*

This week's study showed us how Ruth's love and devotion continued in her efforts to care for Naomi. She was an outsider in a strange land, yet she gained the respect of those with whom she came into contact. She learned about God's love and how He took care of the needs of His people.

You are an heir of God's mercy and love. You must pass those blessings on to others. When you share your own experience and spread the good news of your redeemer, you are passing His blessings on to those who need to know Him.

One way to share God's blessings and love is by quoting Scripture. When you memorize Scripture, you equip yourself with tools to give you more power as you witness to others. God will reveal to you ways to use the tools He has provided in spreading His gospel.

Your First Place program materials give you two resources to help you memorize your memory verse. The Scripture Memory Verses CD can be listened to at home, in the car and while you exercise. Take advantage of them and you will find memorizing much easier. You can take your *Walking in the Word* Scripture memory book with you wherever you go, reading your memory verse whenever you have a spare moment.

The following Scriptures are used as prayers to help you in sharing God's blessings:

Oh, Lord, You have promised that if I delight in You, You will give me the desires of my heart (see Psalm 37:4).

Heavenly Father, You promised to keep me in perfect peace when my mind is steadfast and I trust in You (see Isaiah 26:3).

Lord God, I claim Your promise to meet all my needs according to Your glorious riches in Christ Jesus (see Philippians 4:19).

DAY 7: *Reflections*

The Word of God is true, and it is correct. You read in 2 Timothy 3:16-17 that all Scripture is "God-breathed," or inspired by God. It can be used for reproof as well as teaching, correction and training in righteousness. Charles Stanley wrote, "God is precise in His instruction and promises given through His Word. Meditating upon God's Word is one of the most wonderful ways we can listen to the voice of God for divine guidance."[1]

In your quiet time with Him each day, take time to listen carefully to what God is telling you and where He is leading you. Before accepting anything into your life, filter it through God's Word and eliminate anything that contradicts what the Bible says.

The Word of God is a light for your way, and it illuminates everything so that you will be able to discern truth from fallacy.

Because God's Word is true and powerful in your life, it becomes a weapon to use in your battle against any stronghold that threatens your relationship with God. No matter what your stronghold may be, if it sets itself against God and separates you from Him, it is harmful to you and to your relationship with God.

Be assured that your enemy, Satan, is just waiting for you to stumble into temptation. He works overtime on those who diligently seek God and read His Word. When you couple God's Word with prayer, Satan becomes powerless and flees.

To You, O Lord, I lift up my soul; in You I trust, O my God. Do not let me be put to shame, nor let my enemies triumph over me (see Psalm 25:1-2).[2]

Gird Your sword upon Your side, O Mighty One; clothe Yourself with splendor and majesty. In Your majesty ride forth victoriously in behalf of truth, humility and righteousness; let Your right hand display awesome deeds (see Psalm 45:3-4).[3]

Lord God, I wait for the blessed hope—the glorious appearing of our great God and Savior, Jesus Christ, who gave Himself for us to redeem us from all wickedness and to purify for Himself a people that are His very own, eager to do what is good (see Titus 2:13-14).

Notes
1. Charles Stanley, *In Touch with God* (Nashville, TN: Thomas Nelson, 1997), p. 13.
2. Beth Moore, *Praying God's Word* (Nashville, TN: Broadman and Holman, 2000), p. 318.
3. Ibid., pp. 320-321.

Group Prayer Requests   Today's Date:_____

Name	Request	Results

QUALITIES PLEASING TO GOD

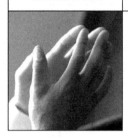

MEMORY VERSE

The LORD does not look at the things man looks at.
Man looks at the outward appearance,
but the LORD looks at the heart.

1 Samuel 16:7

In this week's study, we will observe how the relationship between Ruth and Boaz developed. Their relationship—like any godly love relationship—can give you insight into your love relationship with the Lord. As you study, watch for the character qualities of Ruth and Boaz that are pleasing to the Lord.

DAY 1: *Kindness*

First Place members are encouraged to put Christ in first place in every area of life. As a result of this commitment, we will be able to give more glory to God. Almost everyone wants to be a more attractive person. In today's study, we'll discover that the most attractive traits are not usually physical in nature.

➤ In Ruth 2:4, what does the expression "The LORD be with you" mean to you?

The very first words we hear from Boaz are words of blessing and kindness to the people who worked for him. Sometimes we talk kindly to those who are in authority over us or have higher positions. However, godly kindness knows no level or class. Christ was kind and loving to those with whom He came in contact, especially the poor and children.

Jesus' kindness and consideration attracted the common people of His day. In a similar way, Boaz stood out among the people of his day. He was kind to his servants.

➤ In Ephesians 4:32, what action did Paul suggest as a demonstration of kindness?

➤ Why is kindness linked to forgiveness?

➤ What instruction regarding relationships is given in Proverbs 15:1?

➤ Read Ruth 2:8-9,14. In what ways did Boaz demonstrate kindness toward Ruth?

➤ What words did Naomi use to describe Boaz in verse 20?

As you go about your work this week either at home or on a job, speak kindly to those around you. Showing kindness includes everyone, especially family members. When you have been unkind or hurtful to someone, have you asked for forgiveness? If not, ask God to give you the courage to ask forgiveness from those you may have wronged.

Heavenly Father, give me kind words to say to those with whom I come in contact this week.

Lord, give me the courage to go to those I may have hurt with unkind words in the past and ask for their forgiveness.

DAY 2: *Spirituality*

In Ruth 2:4, the first words spoken by Boaz to his servants were about the Lord. He didn't ask about their work or make a statement about the crops or the weather. Boaz was a spiritual man. He was aware of God's presence in his life. Others were aware of God's presence through his example. The Holy Spirit's presence will shine through you, letting all around you know that you love Christ.

➤ After reading 1 Corinthians 2:13-14, check which of the following Paul indicated is a characteristic of the Spirit-controlled life:

☐ Language

☐ Habits

☐ Appearance

☐ Attitudes

Some people tend to confuse spirituality with attitude. One can have what the world calls a great attitude and have no relationship with God. A person can lead a disciplined life with good habits yet reject Christ. However, discerning God's spirit and expressing spiritual truths in spiritual words cannot be faked by the world.

An important ingredient in spiritual maturity is love, which Jesus said identifies you as His follower.

➤ After reading John 13:34-35, list at least three ways your love can show people you really belong to Christ.

When you choose to give Christ first place in your life, you will surely desire to become more spiritually mature. As you think about the attractiveness of a truly spiritual person, examine your own life. Are you prone to think more about physical or material things than about God and His kingdom? Weight loss and physical conditioning represent worthy goals, but in and of themselves, they do not make a person attractive for the glory of God.

➣ List two or three names of people you know whom you consider to be spiritually mature. Next to each name, write one or two characteristics that indicate that person's spiritual maturity.

Heavenly Father, help me to develop the characteristics of spiritual maturity in my own life.

Thank You, Father God, for sending people into my life to be examples of spiritual maturity for me.

DAY 3: *Physical Appearance*

Do you believe your physical appearance can be an asset to your ability to glorify God? Can it also be a detriment? Improvement of one's physical appearance is not the goal of First Place, but it can be a by-product of commitment to Christ and the First Place program. Remember, the program is not just for losing weight or gaining physical health. You will become a better Christian when you put Christ first in your life.

➣ According to Ruth 2:5-7, what caused Boaz to notice Ruth?

☐ Her character
☐ Her spirituality
☐ Her physical appearance
☐ Her fine jewelry

Because Boaz did not know who the young woman was, he took notice of Ruth. Physical appearance makes the first impression people have of you. For this reason, you can get discouraged easily if you don't look the way you want to look. Lifestyles that include eating right and exercising help you feel better about your appearance.

If you do not achieve your goals as quickly as you would like, remember that pleasing the Lord and obeying Him are more important than reaching a certain weight or size. If you are doing the right things for the right reasons yet not getting the results you want physically, just be patient and know that God will eventually reward your faithfulness.

➤ According to 1 Peter 3:3-4, what is the essence of true beauty? (If you are a man responding to this question, answer in masculine terms.)

➤ What does Proverbs 31:30-31 have to say about the beauty of a woman?

Staying with the First Place program takes patience. It is a complete change of lifestyle and eating habits. This is not a program for several months; it is a program for a lifetime. If you complete the program but return to your old ways of living, you will more than likely gain back any weight lost and neglect the areas of Bible study, prayer and memorizing Scripture. Satan will work overtime to sabotage your efforts. Do not allow discouragement to ruin your efforts to glorify God.

Heavenly Father, grant me the patience to persevere and keep my commitments to You and to the First Place program.

Dear Lord, keep me from being discouraged and help me to continue in my efforts to glorify You at all times.

DAY 4: A Servant's Heart

➤ Boaz may have first noticed Ruth because of her physical attractiveness, but what had he also noticed (Ruth 2:11)?

Boaz had learned that Ruth had a servant's heart. Ruth was working to feed not only herself but Naomi as well. A servant's heart prefers others above self. A servant's heart motivates you to do the work of the Lord for the right reason and in the right way. Christ is our example of humility. He taught us to serve others as a way of serving Him.

➤ Ruth 2:7 describes Ruth's actions as she gleaned that first day. Can you imagine how humbling it must have been to have to pick up leftover grain after the harvesters? What kind of attitude does Ruth seem to display in this situation?

Having a servant's heart becomes increasingly difficult in today's society of selfishness and me-first attitudes. Remember President John F. Kennedy's oft-quoted challenge from his 1961 inauguration: "Ask not what your country can do for you—ask what you can do for your country." Apply that to your Christian service and ask not what others can do for you, but what you can do for others to show your reasonable service and love for Him in return for all that He does give you.

➤ What was Jesus trying to convey to His disciples in Mark 9:35?

➤ In what ways can you serve the Lord unselfishly? In other words, what do you do that does not bring earthly rewards but is motivated by concern for others and your love for God?

You can make a fresh commitment to the Lord to serve Him regardless of the results, recognition or opposition you receive. Seek out opportunities to show your love for God through service to others.

Dear Lord, show me ways that I can serve You and others through my participation in the First Place program.

Heavenly Father, develop in me a true servant's heart so that I may serve You with love every day of my life.

DAY 5: *Diligence*

In Ruth 2:7, another attractive quality of Ruth caught the interest of Boaz. Ruth was also diligent. Diligence means to follow through with your commitments.

➣ What did the foreman tell Boaz about Ruth?

➣ How did Ruth demonstrate her diligence by her actions?

Usually when the gleaners went into the field, they only remained long enough to get grain sufficient for that day, but Ruth worked steadily throughout the day. She fulfilled her commitment and showed her love for Naomi in her diligent efforts to provide for their welfare. She made sure they would have food. In return she was recognized and rewarded greatly.

➣ In 2 Timothy 4:7, how did Paul express the importance of diligence in his own life?

➤ According to 2 Timothy 4:8, what is the reward for such diligence?

➤ Do Paul's words to Timothy express your commitment to continue until you reach your goals?

☐ Yes   ☐ No   ☐ Undecided

➤ On a scale of 1 to 10, rate your level of diligence in staying with the First Place program thus far. This would include attendance at meetings, prayer, Bible reading and study, exercise, following the Live-It Plan and encouraging others in your group. Circle your answer.

1   2   3   4   5   6   7   8   9   10

➤ What are some of the things keeping you from being a 10 in your diligence to fulfill your commitments to First Place?

➤ What could possibly be your earthly rewards for being diligent to follow your commitments to First Place?

Heavenly Father, help me to make a fresh commitment to my efforts in the First Place program so that I may reap a harvest.

Holy Lord, help me to make every effort to be found spotless, blameless and at peace with You

DAY 6: *Reflections*

In this week's study we have learned the characteristics, or qualities, that are pleasing to God. He wants His children to be kind, spiritual, humble and diligent. He wants us to be more willing to serve others than to be served ourselves. He wants our physical appearance to be a reflection of His goodness, grace and love. One way to accomplish, or attain, these qualities in your life is by reading God's Word and using it in your daily life.

Memorized verses can help you in being kind to others and serving them as you think of Scriptures used in this week's study. Ephesians 4:32 is another verse worth memorizing: "Be kind and compassionate to one another, forgiving each other, just as in Christ God forgave you."

Think what this world would be like if every person, not just Christians, practiced this verse. You can remember and repeat it whenever you need to be kind, considerate and compassionate toward others.

In Beth Moore's book *Praying God's Word*, her model of using God's Word when you pray will help you overcome the problems you face daily in your walk with Him.[1] Whether your stronghold is pride, insecurity, rejection, guilt, depression or despair, God will help you overcome it through His powerful words in the Bible.

Heavenly Father, help me to hold fast the confession of my hope without wavering, for He who promised is faithful (see Hebrews 10:23).

Holy God, let me do as You have commanded. Help me to love You, my God, to walk in Your ways and to keep Your commandments (see Deuteronomy 30:16).

Lord Jesus, You have said that I will know that I know You if I keep Your commands, for if I keep Your Word, truly the love of God is perfected in me. By this I can know that I am in You (see 1 John 2:3-5).

Lord God, help me to prepare my mind for action and to be self-controlled; set my hope fully on the grace given me when Jesus revealed Himself to me (see 1 Peter 1:13).

DAY 7: *Reflections*

As a Christian, you are a servant of God. That does not mean you are in bondage as a slave. It means you are a person who chooses to serve the divine master. By doing so you honor Him and His Son, Jesus Christ. As you serve others, you behave in a Christlike manner because Jesus referred to Himself many times as a servant. Just as you emulate Christ as a servant, you want to emulate other characteristics.

Quoting Scripture and prayer are two of those qualities. Jesus quoted the Old Testament many times in his teachings, and prayer was an important part of His lifestyle.

He set up a model prayer for you with the Lord's Prayer in Matthew 6:9-13. He prayed for His disciples and all those who would follow Him when He prayed the intercessory prayer in John 17. He prayed for your protection in verse 15. He prayed for your witness in verse 18. Because God loved you and prayed for you, He expects you to love Him and pray for those who do not know Him.

Jesus demonstrated the importance of prayer in His life when He prayed in the garden of Gethsemane before His death. Over and over again He urged the disciples and His followers to pray in His name. He sought only His Father's will to be done. He knew His Father would answer. Through Jesus' own willing submission to His Father's will, your salvation was bought.

Using Jesus' own words and promises as you pray, demonstrates your great love and devotion to Him. Honoring His name and giving Him glory is an excellent reason for praying God's Word.

Give honor and glory to His name through your prayers and His Word.

"Be exalted, O LORD, in your strength; [I] will sing and praise your might" (Psalm 21:13).

"I will exalt you, O LORD, for you lifted me out of the depths and did not let my enemies gloat over me" (Psalm 30:1).

Praise be to my Lord, to God my Savior, who daily bears my burdens (see Psalm 68:19).

O Lord, I know You do not look at the things that humans look at. Man looks at the outward appearance, but You, O Lord, look at my heart (see 1 Samuel 16:7).

Note
1. Beth Moore, *Praying God's Word* (Nashville, TN: Broadman and Holman, 2000).

GROUP PRAYER REQUESTS   TODAY'S DATE:_____

NAME	REQUEST	RESULTS

PROTECTING YOUR RELATIONSHIP

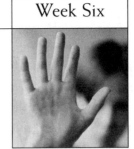

MEMORY VERSE

Submit yourselves, then, to God.
Resist the devil, and he will flee from you.
James 4:7

Ruth and Boaz had to overcome many obstacles to protect and nurture their relationship. They were willing to overcome cultural and racial differences and ignore the prejudices of those around them.

In this week's study, we'll examine our lives to see if we are protecting our relationships with God. Who or what might come between us and our relationship with Him?

DAY 1: *Protect Your Ears*

In Ruth 2:8, Boaz warned Ruth not to listen to others who might want her to glean in their fields. Perhaps Boaz was protecting her from men who would take advantage of her. He may have feared she would be tempted by their offers and perhaps he would lose the possibility of a relationship with her. Thus the first thing he said to her was "listen to me."

In your relationship with the Lord, you must be careful about what you allow to come into your mind through your ears. The ear is the doorstep to the mind, and the mind is the doorstep to the soul.

> ➤ According to Proverbs 2:1-6, to what are you supposed to turn your ear?

➤ From where does wisdom come?

We need to understand that wisdom comes from God. What we hear affects what we think, and what we think determines what we do and who we are. In the computer language of today, a term defines this principle very well. GIGO is actually an acrostic for "garbage in, garbage out." Like a computer, your mind produces garbage if you put garbage into it. Music, for example, can either encourage your spiritual growth or entice you to sinful action.

You must listen to people every day. If people are positive and godly, they will influence you to be the same. If they are negative and worldly, they will influence you in the wrong direction. You must protect your relationship with the Lord by protecting your ears and thus your mind.

➤ What are some of the things that bombard your ears every day?

➤ Some of these you can't control, but others you can. What can you do to control some of the things your ears hear every day?

With all the noise in your daily life, a quiet time of meditation becomes increasingly important. Your quiet time will give you the opportunity to listen for the voice of God and to know Him in a more intimate way.

➤ According to Psalm 34:15b,17, what does God listen to and what does He hear?

God has His ear attuned to you. He listens to your prayers of praise, supplication and thanksgiving. He is aware of what you hear and how you use what you hear in your life. Evaluate what you hear in the light of what is pleasing to Him and what is not.

 Heavenly Father, help me listen for Your voice each day as I read Your Word and help me do what is good and right in Your sight.

Dear Lord, in all the noise that surrounds me each day, may I never cease to listen for Your voice and hear Your instruction for me.

DAY 2: *Protect Your Eyes*

In order to help her glean efficiently, Boaz told Ruth to watch carefully all that was happening in the fields around her. Boaz also gave her a veiled warning to watch out for the men who were harvesting.

➤ What were Boaz's instructions to Ruth in Ruth 2:9? Why did he warn her?

Without a protector, Ruth might have been harassed or victimized by the men. Your eyes are a source of protection, but they are also sources of temptation. The devil enjoys placing before your eyes those things that are your greatest temptations. Images of food appear when you are hungry, images of bed and/or rest appear when you feel too tired to exercise, images of all you have to do appear when you are pressed for time and you haven't done your Bible study. All these images lead you away from God and what He wants for you.

➤ What are three things you see daily that can be temptations?

In order to protect your relationship with the Lord and continue in His blessing, you must learn to protect your eyes. This means staying away from visual images that cause your greatest temptations. Suggestive movies and television shows contain images that can stay in your mind long after the movie or show is over.

➤ After reading 1 Thessalonians 5:22, check the definition that best characterizes the word "avoid."

☐ Frequently partake

☐ Seldom partake

☐ Occasionally partake

☐ Never partake

That's right: it means never partake—stay away from it completely. The very appearance of evil includes visual images that make their way into your mind as tools of Satan to tempt you to disobey the Lord. Are you guarding your eyes?

When you listed areas of temptation you see every day, did you list the newspaper, magazines, television, billboards, store displays and the people around you? Newspapers can tempt you to buy with their enticing ads. Billboards can present images of food that tempt you. The list could go on and on. Satan is busy working overtime to make sure temptation is everywhere.

➤ What are some of the places you as a Christian need to avoid because they promote tempting visual images?

Guard your eyes, so you can continue to live a life that is glorifying to the Lord. Make a commitment to God to avoid places that promote tempting or harmful visual images. Rely on His strength to help you keep this commitment.

 Heavenly Father, guard my eyes as You would my tongue so that they will not be stumbling blocks in my relationship with You.

Lord Jesus, I rely fully on Your strength to help me face temptation daily and keep the commitments I make to You.

DAY 3: *Protect Your Time*

Boaz also warned Ruth to protect her time. He told her to follow his maidens, whom he trusted to lead her in the right direction. By following them, Ruth would successfully glean all that she needed.

A conscious effort is required to focus our time and protect it from trivial things that have no lasting effect.

➤ According to 2 Timothy 2:3-7, what characteristics do the soldier, athlete and farmer have in common?

Focus keeps first things first. Whatever keeps you from focusing on God and His purpose for your life should be gladly omitted from your lifestyle.

➤ What are some activities or responsibilities that may get in the way, robbing you of time?

Many times Christians use busyness as an excuse for not spending time in Bible study, for not giving enough time to prayer or for not exercising and eating healthy.

Plan your day ahead rather than have your time eaten by unplanned events. Someone once said that "to fail to plan is to plan to fail." Is your quiet time for Bible study and prayer a planned part of your schedule? You know it should be, but do you keep putting it off? Think of what you need to do in order for your quiet time to become a daily habit and part of your daily routine.

After reading 1 Corinthians 14:33, complete the following:

God is not a God of_____but of_____.

God is a God of order. If your days are chaotic and wear you out, then you need to look at your planning. Of course things that cause stress and change of routine might happen during the day; but if it seems to happen too frequently, pray about what you need to do to get your life back in order.

Do you tell yourself that when a particular event is over or a project is finished, you will have time to do what you need to do? Then when the project is over or the event is past, you find another project or event takes its place. This happens to many of us.

How many of the excuses you use for not following your commitments to First Place involve time? If most of them do involve time, think about your priorities. Can you organize your time so that you can have a better relationship with the Lord and those closest to you?

Make a list of your priorities for today or tomorrow.

Are these priorities truly important, or are there activities in this list that could be dropped or rescheduled? Remember, plan your work and work your plan. Begin to develop a habit of planning every day before it arrives. Give time to God as your first priority and all of your other activities and responsibilities will fall into place (see Matthew 6:33).

Heavenly Father, help me to plan my time so that I may have more time to spend in Your Word and in prayer.

Lord God, my desire is to please You in all that I do. Show me my priorities and guide me in my daily activities.

DAY 4: *Protect Your Fellowship*

Boaz knew Ruth was more likely to stay in his field if she had a good relationship with the other workers. If you have good fellowship and friendships with those in the church, you are much more likely to stay in right fellowship with the Lord.

➤ What are the five things listed in Colossians 3:12 that we are to clothe ourselves with in our relationships with others?

Just as a lone sheep is more easily devoured by a wolf or lion than a sheep in a flock, Satan wants you out of the church's influence and fellowship. If he can foster unkind, impatient and unforgiving attitudes, his chances multiply greatly.

➤ After reading Hebrews 10:25, check each one of the following in which you participate:

    ☐ Worship service
    ☐ Bible study with a small group (a Sunday School class or weekly study)
    ☐ First Place weekly meeting
    ☐ Home Bible study group meeting
    ☐ Family Bible study

If you are not meeting regularly with a group of Christians for worship and accountability, seek out a group or church.

➤ List the benefits, or blessings, of meeting with a group of Christians on a regular basis for study and worship.

➤ According to 1 Thessalonians 5:11-15, what are some of the things Paul instructed Christians to do one for one another?

Fellowship with other Christians is a vital part of the life of a Christian. That fellowship includes the times when Christians gather for food, fun and games in an atmosphere that promotes good feelings and love for one another. No matter what the occasion, God is pleased when His children gather in His name.

Let your First Place group know you are thankful that God put them in your life to help you grow in Him. Renew your commitment to the group and to fellowshiping with other Christians.

Heavenly Father, thank You for sending other Christians into my life to give me encouragement and prayer when I need it.

Dear Lord, help me to be an encourager and a prayer warrior for those with whom I fellowship. Help me to be sensitive to their needs.

DAY 5: *Protect Your Strength*

Relationships require energy! They cannot run smoothly without regard for physical stamina and good health.

➤ According to Ruth 2:9,14, how did Boaz seek to meet Ruth's physical needs?

Caring for your body reflects appreciation for our creator who designed us to need healthy food and water.

Although bad things happen to good people, the possibilities of health and well-being increase as you lead a healthy lifestyle and live in harmony with God's teachings. Your participation in a First Place group provides tools to help you in the areas of food and exercise. The First Place Commitment Record, or CR, gives you a place to keep a record of what you are doing in the First Place program.

➤ According to Philippians 1:20, what did Paul want for his body?

➤ How can God be exalted through your body?

➤ What did Paul tell the people at Corinth about their bodies in 1 Corinthians 6:17-20?

Is there anything about your lifestyle that might be harmful to your body? Pray about how you can cleanse your body and honor God.

You must never leave yourself unprotected from temptation, as Hank, a First Place member discovered firsthand. As a new member, Hank won the battle against overeating during the Christmas holidays. In fact, he even lost weight. However, when January and February came, Hank gained back all he had lost because he let down his guard. Remember, God will provide the means to escape temptations when you seek His help.

➤ What is the wonderful promise found in 1 Corinthians 10:13?

Heavenly Father, I claim Your promise today that You will provide a way for me to resist the temptations that come into my life.

Thank You, Father God, for giving me the means to protect my strength. May I always exalt and honor You with my body.

DAY 6: *Reflections*

Protecting your physical strength is important to God, but the protection of your mind and heart are equally important. The Bible study this week emphasized the importance of protecting your eyes, your ears, your fellowship and your time. God provides all the protection you need through the sword of the Spirit and prayer. Against these two, even Satan loses power (see Ephesians 6:10-11).

Scripture memory strengthens your mind and spirit. You fill your mind with thoughts of God and what He has done for you and the power He has to do even more. Each study challenges you with 10 verses to memorize and make a part of your life. Your leaders are committed to memorizing them too. They will help you and encourage you in all your endeavors as a member of a First Place group.

Use the Scripture memory CD and *Walking in the Word* book to help you seal the words of the memory verses in your heart and mind. You will be reminded of these resources each week either through the days of reflection or by your leaders. Take advantage of them.

You have also learned about using Scripture in prayer. The use of God's Word and prayer together give you strength to overcome any stronghold.

"Do not withhold Your mercy from me, O LORD, may your love and your truth always protect me" (Psalm 40:11).

O Lord, You have promised to protect me and preserve my life. You will bless me in the land and will not surrender me to my foes (see Psalm 41:2).

Heavenly Father, You are faithful and I rely on You to strengthen me and protect me from the evil one (see 2 Thessalonians 3:3).

DAY 7: *Reflections*

One of the most precious prayers found in God's Word is the prayer Jesus prayed for the disciples and all Christians to come. This prayer is found in John 17. To know that our Lord and Savior prayed to His Father on our behalf is amazing. In John 17:15, He particularly prayed for our protection "from the evil one." Take time to read the entire chapter. You will see how much God cares for you. In the face of His own death, He took the time to pray for His disciples and all those who would come after Him.

With Jesus setting the example, you have even more reason to strengthen your own prayer time. One of the most effective ways to do this is use Scriptures in your prayers. After memorizing the 10 verses for this study, you will have a base on which to add other verses you find to memorize.

You will find that the more you study God's Word, the more you will want to memorize it. Some of the verses become so important to you that you can't imagine not having them and using them.

In the remaining weeks of this study, work on your commitments to the program and memorize the verses, if you have not done so already. At the end of the study, volunteer to say all 10 aloud to your leader or to your group. The more Scripture you find to memorize, the more power you have to battle Satan and overcome temptation. Pray and seek God's help with memorizing His Word; He is faithful and will reward your efforts in His name.

The following Scripture prayers are taken from Psalms. In this book you will find words of praise, thanksgiving, supplication and confession. This would be a good place to start with memorizing Scriptures in addition to the memory verse for the week.

"Give ear to my words, O LORD, consider my sighing. Listen to my cry for help, my King and my God, for to you I pray" (Psalm 5:1).

Lord God, "may the words of my mouth and the meditation of my heart be pleasing in your sight, O LORD, my Rock and my Redeemer" (Psalm 19:14).

Father, I submit myself to You. Help me to resist the devil, so he will flee from me (see James 4:7).

GROUP PRAYER REQUESTS   TODAY'S DATE:_____

NAME	REQUEST	RESULTS

IN GOD'S HANDS

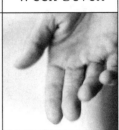

MEMORY VERSE

My God will meet all your needs according to his glorious riches in Christ Jesus.

Philippians 4:19

As a Christian, you receive wonderful care from the loving hand of God. This week's study will reveal much about the hands of the Lord and your proper response to His care. You will see how God supplies all the needs in your life.

DAY 1: *Jealous Hands*

In Exodus 20:5, God described Himself as "a jealous God." His jealousy is not the possessive kind that wants someone selfishly for what he or she can get. Rather, God is jealous for you. He wants the best for you and protects you from false gods by commanding you to worship Him alone.

Humans quite normally want to look out for the safety of those they care about. Although Ruth was a stranger to Boaz, his compassion prompted him to protect her.

➤ After reading Ruth 2:8, why do you think Boaz didn't want Ruth to glean in fields other than his?

➤ In Ruth 2:22, why did Naomi agree with Boaz's advice?

≫ Was Boaz jealous of Ruth or for Ruth? Why do you think so?

≫ What did Boaz tell Ruth in Ruth 2:9?

Boaz was concerned about Ruth's safety. The human desire to protect comes from God, the ultimate protector. As you studied last week, a child of God living in the will of God receives protection by His hand.

≫ In 2 Corinthians 11:2, Paul mentions "godly jealousy"; what do you think he meant by this type of jealousy (see Ephesians 5:25-27)?

≫ In Psalm 5:11, what are those who take refuge in the Lord to do?

Always remember this: God protects you because He loves you.

≫ How does Paul describe love in 1 Corinthians 13:7?

≫ How does that description of godly love affect you?

≫ Describe a time when you have felt God's hands of protection on your life. Have you thanked Him for His protection?

Lord God, show me the way I can put You first always in my life.

Thank You, Heavenly Father, for Your protection and love for me.

DAY 2: *Praising Hands*

God's care and love for His children gives every Christian reason to praise God. He imparts that love to you with a kindness that only He can give, just as Boaz showed kindness to Ruth.

≫ According to Ruth 2:10,13, how did Ruth feel about Boaz's kindness to her?

Just as Ruth responded to Boaz's concern for her welfare and safety with gratitude and humility, so should Christians respond to God's loving-kindness with the same attitude.

The position that Ruth assumed—bowing down with her face to the ground—is the posture of worship. Your response to God's grace should include sincere worship. A significant part of worship is praise.

≫ List some of the reasons you want to praise God.

➤ According to Psalm 9:1-2, how did David praise God?

David praised God through the psalms he wrote. Psalms 34:1-10; 40:1-5 and 103:1-5 give some of the reasons David praised God. Look them up and read them. Mark them and reread them often to remind you of God's loving care for you—especially when you are feeling down, or discouraged.

Examine your own heart. Are you able to praise God with a humble heart? Are you "bowed down" with gratitude for His blessings? Consider the reasons for praising God that you listed above, and give Him thanks for His love.

 Heavenly Father, thank You for taking care of me and filling all my needs through Your Son, Christ Jesus.

Lord God, help me to continually bow down and praise Your holy name in all that I do.

DAY 3: *Providing Hands*

As an outsider, Ruth had no privileges. She wasn't even supposed to be allowed to glean in the fields. Boaz saw her need and her devotion to Naomi, and he acted in kindness toward her and provided for her.

➤ According to Ruth 2:14-15, how did Boaz take care of Ruth at mealtime?

The only people usually allowed to participate in the meal prepared for the workers were those who were members of the owner's family. Thus Ruth received immediate treatment as a family member. By custom, she should have been rejected even from gleaning, but here she sat at the master's table.

God does amazing things and provides for you daily. You don't deserve the love and the care He provides—no one does. Everyone was a sinner and an outsider until Jesus came and provided the means for each person to come to His table.

≫ In verse 14, what did Boaz give Ruth to eat?

Some interpret this action to mean that Boaz fed Ruth from his own hand. She is not only allowed to glean and sit at the dinner table, but she is also fed by the master's hand. The person who deserved it least, but needed it most, was given the greatest gift possible.

Just as Ruth, when you were a stranger, or foreigner, and deserved to be exiled from God and all His blessings, He reached down to you in grace. The master gave you food from heaven—Jesus, the Bread of Life—and made you His own. You deserve the least and get the most. This is grace! God treats you as a family member. Isn't that amazing?

≫ Consider Ephesians 2:11-14. How do you feel about being accepted into God's family?

Catherine joined First Place to help combat the effects of diabetes. She had grown up as a foster child and never had a family of her own. In First Place, she experienced the joy of a caring group. Catherine often called her group her family. Later when Catherine became a Christian and joined a church, her family grew to include new brothers and sisters in Christ. Now Catherine leads a First Place group. She says, "I ask God to lead people to my group who need a sense of belonging. There is always room in my family for one more."

In First Place, you will learn that you are accepted by God, even when you feel unaccepted or unworthy. He sees you in a different light. Although Jesus sees you at your worst, He died to make you His best. His hand of provision is working in your life to make you all you can be. Review the memory verse for this week. Believe that God will provide for you and do amazing things, just as Boaz took care of Ruth.

As you go through the day, encourage others and tell someone how blessed you are to be a child of God.

 Heavenly Father, I sing a song of thanksgiving to You and praise Your name for Your wonderful provision for me.

Lord God, I want to be my best for You because You sent Your beloved Son to die for me, and I am now a redeemed child of God.

DAY 4: *Working Hands*

After Ruth humbly thanked Boaz for his kindness in Ruth 2:13, she simply ate and then went to work! Ruth could have waited around to see what else Boaz might give her. She might have played helpless in hopes of getting handouts from the servant girls. She could have complained about the heat or asked for the day off. Instead, Ruth quickly got up to glean.

➣ After reading Genesis 2:2; John 5:17 and Hebrews 7:24-25, answer the following questions:

Does God work?   ☐ Yes   ☐ No

Does Jesus work?   ☐ Yes   ☐ No

➣ What work is Jesus doing right now?

When you stop to think about your life, you realize that God is always at work in some way to make your life better or to help you grow in Him. When He sends times of testing, or trial, you might wish God wouldn't work so hard. Jesus worked on Earth to bring understanding to His followers, and He continues His work in heaven through the Holy Spirit in your life. You are created in God's image, and He expects you to work to know Him more intimately.

Some think of the First Place commitments as work. In essence they may be work, and at the beginning, they are certainly hard work. Just as any job becomes easier with the experience of doing it, however, your First Place commitments will become easier as you make them a part of your life. Seek to make them a lifestyle habit, and they will not be overwhelming but rather a normal part of your weekly routine.

➤ How does Colossians 3:17 apply to what you do every day?

As you work today, work for the Lord's sake as though He were your employer. Tell Him you are doing this because you love Him.

 Lord Jesus, help me today to remember Your great love for me and to give thanks to You in everything I do.

Heavenly Father, let everything I do in word or deed today bring praise and honor to Your name through Christ Jesus.

DAY 5: *Purposeful Hands*

Boaz was not content to leave it to chance that Ruth would pick up sufficient grain on her own.

➤ According to Ruth 2:15-16, what did Boaz tell his harvesters to do?

➤ In verses 17-20, what did Naomi notice about the amount of grain Ruth brought back? Why did she bless Boaz?

By instructing his harvesters to purposefully leave some grain behind, Boaz was insuring that Naomi and Ruth would have more than just the bare minimum. All through the Bible you find examples of God's blessings. He is not simply generous; He is extravagant in His giving.

Joshua told the people of Israel that God would do amazing things for them when they consecrated themselves to Him (see Joshua 3:5). "Consecrating" means to clean and prepare for maximum use. You must be consecrated to the Lord for His use. Do you have areas of your life the Holy Spirit wants to cleanse, but you refuse to yield to Him? Are you allowing God to use First Place to teach you how to be controlled by His Spirit in every aspect of your life? Resolve today to let God have control in every area of your life. You will find your life to be better and fuller when He is in control. God will fill you to overflowing with blessings that will amaze you.

Read 2 Kings 4:1-7 to see the amazing way God provided for a poor widow.

➤ Why did God provide for the widow's needs?

➤ How did God provide for the need?

The widow cried out to Elisha, a man of God, and asked for help. You must ask before you expect to receive. In Matthew 6:11, Jesus gives the disciples a model prayer. In it is included the line "Give us today our daily bread." He will provide when you ask.

➤ What is the promise found in Matthew 7:7-8?

➤ Have you claimed that promise? Briefly describe an answered prayer or how God provided for you in an amazing way.

If you have a need you feel has gone unmet, ask God for His generous help. If God does not answer your prayer quickly, ask yourself what His purpose might be in delay.

➤ What might He want to teach you while you wait?

Steve joined First Place because he had witnessed the change in the life of his wife, Janet, through her participation in the program. Janet not only lost weight, but she was walking closer to God, enjoying a personal relationship with her Savior. At first, Steve lost weight quickly through the program; but then he reached a plateau. Even though he was frustrated and impatient with this delay, Steve completed the session. Later he told his group, "If I had lost all the weight in the first few months, I would have quit. Then I wouldn't have developed the discipline of a daily quiet time. I'm so glad God didn't grant my request immediately!"

Perhaps you are like Steve. Don't feel discouraged. God is still working—His timetable is simply different from yours. Accept the blessings He does give and renew your efforts in the program.

➤ What is the glorious message of Joshua 23:14?

➤ How does this verse apply to your efforts in First Place?

God will keep His promises because He is a faithful God. You can count on Him!

Thank You, Father, for the great and amazing things You plan to show me when I consecrate my life to You.

Lord God, help me to remember Your promises to me and claim those promises every day as I serve You.

DAY 6: *Reflections*

In this week's study we learned about the many ways God can do amazing things for us. He first asks us to consecrate ourselves. As we prepare ourselves for His maximum use, we rid our lives of anything that hinders and sins which so easily entangle us. Anything that prevents us from being fully ready for God's use is a stronghold. Strongholds become idols which take us away from God. In *Praying God's Word*, Beth Moore explains that until we turn from our idols to the one true God, we will never find liberty, for freedom comes from the Spirit of the Lord.[1]

It is in our own weakness that God is made strong. He gives us His Word coupled with our prayers to use as a weapon to overcome our strongholds. In Jeremiah 29:13, we read that if we seek Him with all our heart, we will find Him.

Indeed, if you seek God in His Word, you *will* find Him. Use God's Word as a weapon against your stronghold, and you will be victorious.

The best way to make God's Word your own is to memorize it and use it in times of stress, temptation and difficulties. God's Word never fails you. When you have a number of verses memorized, you have a resource and a weapon mightier than any situation than you could possibly face.

Lord God, You promised to be near me and that I would find You if I seek You with all my heart. Lord, I seek You now and claim Your promise (see Jeremiah 29:13).

Holy Lord, You have said You will keep me in perfect peace when my mind is stayed on You and I trust in You. Grant me that peace, Lord (see Isaiah 26:3).

Oh, Father, how I thank You that my help comes from You, the maker of heaven and Earth (see Psalm 121:2).[2]

DAY 7: *Reflections*

Once you accept Christ and become a child of the King, He will never abandon you. It is you who strays from God. He is always ready to listen to your prayers and give you comfort. It is up to you to return when you stray or neglect spending time with God.

The Scriptures instruct you to take captive every thought to make it obedient to Christ (see 2 Corinthians 10:5). Beth Moore says that we take our thoughts captive and make them obedient to Christ "every time we choose to think Christ's thoughts about any situation or stronghold instead of Satan's or our own."[3] How will you know what Christ thinks? Read God's Word and you will know what and how Christ thinks. Sounds simple? It is when you gird up your mind and strengthen it with Scripture you have memorized.

Prayer using Scripture as a base brings you into intimate communication with God, and your mind is renewed and strengthened. Scripture memory takes time and diligence, but it can be one of the most rewarding times you spend in God's Word. You have a music CD and the *Walking in the Word* book in your First Place materials to help you. If you are keeping a prayer journal, write the verse in it and repeat it every day. With *Walking in the Word* in front of you, you can repeat the verse each day as you study. Remember, the more times you say a verse or write a verse, the more in-grained it becomes. You write it on your heart where it becomes a part of you.

You, my God, have put Your words in my mouth and covered me with the shadow of Your hand—You who set the heavens in place, who laid the foundations of the earth and who say to Zion, "You are my people" (see Isaiah 51:16).[4]

O, Lord my God, help me never to worship any other god, for You, my Lord, are a jealous God (see Exodus 20:4-5).[5]

My Father, help me to know that You, the Lord my God, is God; You are the faithful God, keeping Your covenant of love to a thousand generations of those who love You and keep Your commands (see Deuteronomy 7:9).[6]

Father, thank You for meeting all my needs through the glorious riches of Christ Jesus (see Philippians 4:19).

Notes

1. Beth Moore, *Praying God's Word* (Nashville, TN: Broadman and Holman, 2000), p. 20.
2. Ibid., p. 25.
3. Ibid., p. 7.
4. Ibid., p. 27.
5. Ibid., p. 28.
6. Ibid.

GROUP PRAYER REQUESTS   TODAY'S DATE:_____

NAME	REQUEST	RESULTS

PREPARING FOR GOD'S BEST

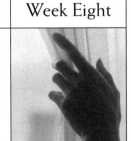

MEMORY VERSE
Joshua told the people, "Consecrate yourselves,
for tomorrow the LORD will do amazing
things among you."
Joshua 3:5

If you knew you were going to meet an important person who would have
a lot of influence over your future, how would you prepare? Ruth's preparation for her meeting with Boaz can teach you much about preparing for
blessings from God. In this week's study, look for attitudes and actions that
reflect readiness on your part to let God supply your needs.

DAY 1: *Don't Settle for Less*

The memory verse this week is a reminder of how God does amazing
things for those who consecrate themselves to Him. Let's see how He
took care of Ruth's needs in an amazing way.

➺ According to Ruth 3:1-2, why did Naomi play matchmaker for Ruth?

➺ Why did Naomi consider Boaz a suitable marriage partner (see 2:20)?

Naomi knew Boaz was a kinsman of the family, though Ruth was
unaware of this fact that first day she went to glean. Naomi probably also
recognized the potential for a wonderful relationship with Boaz because

of his generosity and kindness to Ruth. She believed Boaz was God's best marriage partner for Ruth.

How often are you willing to wait for God's best in your life? Do you settle for second place or less because it takes less time, patience and discipline?

⋙ What is the great promise in Jeremiah 29:11-12?

⋙ What plans do you think God has for you?

⋙ What is the promise found in Jeremiah 33:3?

⋙ Why should you trust God's plans for you?

When Joan joined First Place, she had never heard of Matthew 6:33, which refers to seeking God's will—and not our own—for our lives. Soon after she joined the program, Joan was offered a promotion in her company. Although the job offered more money, she did not think the job description fit her. Remembering Matthew 6:33, Joan prayed for God's best and felt led to turn down the promotion, even though her coworkers thought she had made a mistake. Three months later, a classified ad describing Joan's dream job appeared in the paper. Joan applied for and got the job—because she asked God for His best!

Pray for God to lead you in facing decisions in the future. Ask Him to lead you to do your best and ask Him for protection from the temptation to settle for less than He is willing to supply.

Heavenly Father, help me to always depend on You for all my needs.

Lord, thank You for caring about me and leading me in the direction I should take for my life.

DAY 2: *Do Your Spiritual Homework*

Naomi believed Boaz was God's best choice of a husband for Ruth. However, she did not send an unprepared Ruth out to meet him.

⟫ What were the instructions given to Ruth by Naomi in Ruth 3:3?

Just as Naomi told Ruth to cleanse herself before meeting Boaz, we must be cleansed before we can receive God's best. Spiritual cleansing comes into our lives for the first time at salvation. Few people like to move into an unclean house. The Lord Himself always cleanses us spiritually when He comes into our lives.

⟫ Read Titus 3:4-7. Why are we incapable of cleansing ourselves?

If we were capable of righteous acts, Christ's sacrifice on the cross would have been unnecessary. Praise God for His mercy! Christ's righteousness covers our unrighteousness. Once we are clean through salvation, we adorn ourselves with the clothing of righteousness.

⟫ In several places the Bible mentions being clothed in righteousness (see Job 29:14; Isaiah 61:10; Zechariah 3:3-5; Ephesians 6:14; Revelation 19:8). What does it mean to be clothed in righteousness?

In addition to clothing ourselves with righteousness, we need to confess our sin and live a holy life pleasing to God.

 Heavenly Father, take control of my life and lead me to follow Your will daily.

Lord Jesus, thank You for Your mercy and for the righteousness of Christ which covered my sins on the cross.

DAY 3: *Exercise Faith*

Don't forget: Ruth had a choice about whether or not to follow Naomi's advice. She may have found Naomi's instructions strange and unfamiliar, probably different from the customs of her own country. Besides, Naomi was old and perhaps out of touch with modern society. Fortunately, Ruth had faith in Naomi. She trusted Naomi's counsel. Ruth was later rewarded for her faith when Boaz agreed to take his role as her kinsman-redeemer. God will reward your faith when you call on Him to supply your needs.

➳ What is the promise found in 1 John 5:4-5?

➳ What gives you the victory and power to overcome the world?

In verse 4 the Greek word for "faith" implies action. Real faith reaches out and takes hold of something tangible. It is not just a belief in your head but a belief causing you to act on what you know to be true.

➳ What is the definition of "faith" as found in Hebrews 11:1?

Naomi took action on her faith after God had shown her His plan for Ruth's future. As God shows you His will for each day, you must lay hold of all those things God intends for you to have. If He supplies your needs but you don't make use of them, you miss a blessing.

➤ What are the action words used in 1 Timothy 6:12?

Just as Ruth had to trust Naomi, you must trust God to know what is best for you. The memory verse reminds you that God supplies all your needs. Although your expectation or definition of needs may not be the same as God's, you know He is trustworthy and will give you what you need.

Heavenly Father, give me the faith I need to trust You with any problem or need in my life.

Lord God, give me the opportunity today to share my faith with others.

DAY 4: *Act in Obedience*

After you have spiritually prepared for a significant action or change, you demonstrate your faith by taking action. Otherwise, you cannot claim what is yours from the Lord. Just as Ruth could have dressed in her finest and then stayed home or not done what Naomi instructed, you can prepare yourself for the Lord's work and never act on what you know to do.

➤ According to Ruth 3:5-6, to what extent was Ruth willing to follow Naomi's instruction?

➤ In which of the following areas do you have the most difficulty with consistency in your daily walk of righteousness? Check those that apply.

- ☐ Devotional life
- ☐ Thought life
- ☐ Temper
- ☐ Patience
- ☐ Attitude
- ☐ Habits
- ☐ Appetite
- ☐ Marriage/family
- ☐ Words

You can prepare and have faith that God will bless you, but if you don't have the spirit of obedience, you will reach a stopping place and go no further than your disobedience. God always builds into every victory an obedience test before the final doorway to victory.

➤ According to Genesis 22:2, how did God test Abraham's faith?

You can read the rest of the story of Abraham and Isaac in Genesis 22. You will also see faith in the lives of Moses and David and the other great heroes of the Bible as you read the Old Testament. A roll call of these men who proved their faith is found in Hebrews 11. Sadly enough, many Christians turn back at the point of the obedience test and never reach the pinnacle of faith.

God's obedience test is never intended for Him to find out about your heart. He knows your heart better than you do. The obedience test shows you something about yourself. Whether your test concerns your eating habits, your prayer life or other daily habits, do whatever He says and nothing less and you will succeed.

≫ After reading John 14:21, describe how you believe your love for Christ is being tested through your commitment to change your lifestyle.

After Martha had been a First Place leader for several years, job and family commitments kept her from serving for a while. However, she continued to feel God leading her back to her place of leadership. She reasoned she didn't have time to teach the Bible study properly and, rather than not doing it well, she'd rather not do it at all. Finally, she could resist God no longer and volunteered for a session. A day or two later she received a call asking if she minded having a coleader who wanted to teach the Bible study but didn't feel as good about teaching the food part. Because Martha remained obedient to God's call, He provided a way for her to be faithful to her commitment. He provided for her need.

God will never require of you more than you are able to give. Watch for attitudes, thoughts or actions that hinder your obedience. When you recognize one, begin to pray immediately for strength to overcome it and continue in your pursuit of holiness.

≫ Was there a time in your life when you followed God's will instead of your own and He fulfilled your needs with a greater blessing because of it? Briefly describe what happened.

Heavenly Father, help me to always be open and obedient to Your call of service or sacrifice.

Lord God, give me the strength to overcome my weaknesses so that I may continue my pursuit of holiness.

DAY 5: Claim the Blessing

➤ After reading Ruth 3:7-18, describe how Boaz rewarded Ruth's efforts in verse 15.

Ruth could have protested that she did not deserve God's blessings. She could have felt unworthy of Boaz's attention. She could have refused the barley grain out of false pride. Instead, Ruth claimed her blessings!

➤ Are there great blessings of God you have wanted to claim for yourself but did not feel worthy of accepting?

☐ Yes   ☐ No

Imagine entering the gates of heaven and seeing the Lord for the first time. As you walk down the gold-paved streets, you find yourself inside one of the largest structures in all of heaven. As you look around, you see displayed on the wall of this magnificent mansion wonderful trophies of all the things you had ever hoped for in this lifetime. When you ask the Lord what it all means, He replies, "These are all the blessings I had waiting for you. Some you never asked me for, and some you asked me for but never claimed."

➤ Although this scene is simply imaginary, does it suggest a life principle you may need to adopt? Write the principle and share it with your group at the next meeting.

➤ What are some of the ways God has met your needs?

⤳ Were there times when He supplied more than you actually needed? Briefly describe these times.

In light of how God meets your needs abundantly, how can you claim those things you have asked for in His name but never fully received? Have you called to Him to show you the great and unsearchable things you don't know about? When He shows you those things, listen carefully and follow His instructions obediently.

 Father God, I claim Your promises and blessings today. Help me to see any sin that may be in the way of my receiving Your fullest blessings.

Thank You, Father, for Your willingness to forgive my sin when I ask for and seek Your mercy.

DAY 6: *Reflections*

In this week's study you have learned the importance of preparing for God's best. Faith and obedience are two components of that preparation. Your faith can be strengthened through God's Word. He will show you the importance of being obedient to His will for your life and how to be obedient.

As last week's memory verse says, "God will meet all your needs." One way He meets, or provides for, your need is through the Bible. God's Word has the answers for whatever temptation, obstacle, attitude or need comes your way. When you have a storehouse of memory verses for the different aspects of your life, you have all you need to fight your battle against Satan.

Beth Moore's book *Praying God's Word* gives examples of hundreds of Scriptures to use in your prayer life. Beth writes that she doesn't use Scripture every time she prays because she doesn't "always pray any certain way, but I can confidently tell you this: I have never discovered a more powerful way to demolish strongholds in my life than praying Scripture. When it comes to warfare, this approach is without question the one I most often apply."[1]

Take advantage of God's supply of Scripture, and arm yourself with the two things Satan cannot withstand: prayer and God's Word. Like Ruth, you must be prepared and go forward and claim the blessings God will supply. What greater blessing can you have than to overcome an obstacle, or stronghold, in your life and draw closer to God? Claim His promise today.

Father God, make me strong and courageous. Help me not to be afraid or terrified because of anyone else, for You, the Lord my God, will never leave or forsake me (see Deuteronomy 31:6).

Lord, how I thank You for the assurance that You will not reject Your people; You will never forsake Your inheritance (see Psalm 94:14).

How I thank You, Lord, for having the power to turn any curse into a blessing for me because You, the Lord my God, love me (see Deuteronomy 23:5).

DAY 7: *Reflections*

No one wants to settle for less than the best that life has to offer, but many do just that. They are content with just getting by when with a little effort they can have a better life. In the Christian life this means that many go along in life believing in the Son of God as their personal Savior, but they don't know Him intimately as their best friend. They settle for being an acquaintance but not a close friend. They know about God's blessings, His riches, His love and His mercy, but they don't spend daily time with Him in prayer and Bible study. They miss out on the greater measure He gives to those who call on His name and seek His face.

Your best friend is one to whom you can turn and on whom you can count for support when problems arise or when overwhelming things happen to you. That best friend listens and prays for you. My friend, God is closer to you than even a best friend. He provides that earthly person to give you support here. God gives you support when you feel all else has failed and you feel alone. God never leaves you alone. He sent the Holy Spirit to dwell in you for comfort, peace, guidance and love.

One of the memory verses from another study in First Place talks about a God of hope who will "fill you with all joy and peace as you trust in him, so that you may overflow with hope by the power of the Holy Spirit" (Romans 15:13). What a tremendous promise!

Review what you have learned from other days of reflection concerning memorizing Scripture and remember, no task is too great or difficult for you when you approach it one day at a time. Only two more weeks remain in this study. Make the best use of that time and spend it with God. He will give you the endurance and perseverance you need to finish your race.

 Father, continue to bring me along so that I can rejoice in my sufferings because I know that suffering produces perseverance (see Romans 5:3).

"May your unfailing love be my comfort, according to your promise to your servant. Let your compassion come to me that I may live, for your law is my delight. My soul faints with longing for your salvation, but I have put my hope in Your word" (Psalm 119:76-77,81).

"In You, O LORD, I have taken refuge; let me never be put to shame; deliver me in your righteousness. Turn your ear to me, come quickly to my rescue; be my rock of refuge, a strong fortress to save me" (Psalm 31:1-2).

Heavenly Father, I consecrate myself to You, for tomorrow You will do amazing things for me (see Joshua 3:5).

Note
1. Beth Moore, *Praying God's Word* (Nashville, TN: Broadman and Holman, 2000), p. 8.

GROUP PRAYER REQUESTS   TODAY'S DATE:_____

NAME	REQUEST	RESULTS

STANDING ON THE PROMISES

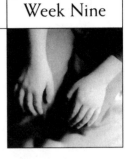

MEMORY VERSE

My dear brothers, stand firm. Let nothing move you. Always give yourselves fully to the work of the Lord, because you know that your labor in the Lord is not in vain.

1 Corinthians 15:58

The winds of adversity often blow hardest just before the greatest victory. In the final chapter of Ruth you get a glimpse of how Boaz, Ruth and Naomi handled adversity by faith. In this week's study, their example will help you to stand firm through difficulties until you reach the place of blessing God has for you.

DAY 1: *Standing in the Gate*

In last week's study, Boaz expressed his willingness to fulfill the responsibility of the kinsman-redeemer and marry Ruth. However, an obstacle was in his path. Another family member was the nearest of kin and had the first right to redeem the property and marry Ruth.

In Ruth 4:1-4, we can read how Boaz handled the situation. He first went to the city gate where legal matters were settled and public decisions were announced.

➳ In verses 1 and 2, why did Boaz wait at the town gate?

➳ Why did he invite the 10 elders too?

Boaz immediately addressed the matter of redeeming the property of Elimelech's family.

➤ In verse 4, what was the closest kinsman-redeemer willing to do?

➤ What was this kinsman-redeemer unwilling to do according to verse 6?

Notice that Boaz did not hide, misrepresent or manipulate the situation. He did not take the other man aside and persuade him in private. He sought the wise counsel of others. Just as Boaz followed the proper procedures and went through the proper channels to settle the matter that faced him, you should seek to model Christian business practices with everyone you encounter.

No matter whether you are employed away from home, retired or staying at home to care for your family, you come into contact with people with whom you do business. Are you guilty of sometimes seeking your own good at the expense of someone else?

➤ What are some of the ways you can be a Christian example in your everyday encounters with people?

Heavenly Father, guide me as I make decisions today so that I will honor You in everything I do.

Father God, help me to wisely seek the counsel of those You place in my life for the purpose of giving me guidance.

DAY 2: *Standing with Experience*

In Ruth 4:3, you learn that Naomi was willing to sell Elimelech's land to the kinsman-redeemer. The piece of land was all Naomi had in the world. When she sold it to the kinsman-redeemer, she would become his property along with the land she sold him. When you give your life to Christ, you become the property of Christ. He is your redeemer. He is the one who cares for you because you belong to Him.

Experience had taught Naomi that she could trust both God and her kinsman-redeemer to take care of her. However, trusting God and others was not an easy decision for Naomi.

➤ Consider Ruth 1:20-21; 2:20; 3:18. Can you see the progression of Naomi's faith? What obstacles did Naomi have to overcome in order to exercise her faith?

Can you imagine the moments Naomi and Ruth spent waiting for Boaz to return? Did they pace anxiously or go about their business as usual? Ruth 3:18 hints that Naomi calmed Ruth by reminding her that Boaz would take care of everything—a picture of what our kinsman-redeemer does for us.

➤ How does 1 Peter 5:6-7 relate to Naomi's experience?

➤ What were some of the concerns that brought you to First Place?

➤ Through goal setting and the commitments of First Place, what have you learned in relation to your concerns?

➤ What is the promise of 1 Peter 5:7?

As you look back on the experiences you have had with the Lord in the past eight weeks, do you find He has sustained you? Cast all your cares on Him. He is faithful and will care for you. Visualize handing Christ your worries. Place them safely in His loving hands. Now you can go through the remainder of the day aware that He is taking care of you.

 Dear God, I hand all my worries and anxieties over to Your loving care. I know You will sustain me and care for me because You love me. Help me not to try to take my cares back from You!

Thank You, Father God, for being the One in whom I can trust and to whom I can give my life.

DAY 3: *Standing at All Costs*

When Naomi's nearest of kin heard she had a piece of land to be claimed, he agreed to fulfill the role of kinsman-redeemer. He stood to gain financially from the circumstances. However, when he heard that a childless widow and children to raise in the name of her deceased husband were included, he lost interest and gave them over to Boaz.

➤ Considering Ruth 4:6, why was the kinsman-redeemer unwilling to marry Ruth?

Like so many people who do not live by faith, the nearest kinsman missed a wonderful opportunity to do the will of the Lord and become a major part of biblical history. He let an opportunity pass because it would complicate his inheritance. He no doubt had children who would not want to share their father's wealth with other offspring. The price was too high for him to pay.

Are you willing to stand at all costs to do the will of the Lord? Will you pay the price and glorify the Lord through your obedience, or will you pass up a wonderful opportunity because you think the price is too high?

➽ Read the story in Matthew 19:16-30 about the rich young man who questioned Jesus concerning how to gain eternal life. What must we be willing to give up to follow Jesus?

➽ What do you prize above everything else in your life?

➽ Is there anything listed that you would place above Christ in your life?

What could be more valuable than following Christ and having eternal life? Christ never intended for you to forsake your family or neglect providing for them. However, He does want to be first place in your life. If you do find any person, place or thing becoming more important than your time with God, confess it to Him. Give Him first place in all that you do today.

Father, thank You for Your redeeming grace—grace I don't deserve. Help me to put You first in my life.

Lord Jesus, help me today to do everything I do in Your name and to bring honor and glory to Your name.

DAY 4: *Standing with Honor*

In Ruth 4:7, you learn more about some rather odd customs of ancient Israel. Men treated each other with honor and respect in their business dealings in an unusual way.

➣ According to Ruth 4:7, what was the custom for finalizing the transfer of property in that time?

➣ What did the kinsman say and do in verse 8?

After the near kinsman declined the privilege of redeeming the land and marrying Ruth, he handed his sandal to Boaz as a sign that Boaz had the right to perform the role himself. Most scholars believe this was their way of closing the deal, much like a signature on a legal document. You will find this custom also mentioned in Deuteronomy 25:8-10.

➣ According to the ancient law, was this an action of honor or dishonor?

➣ According to the Deuteronomy passage, was the one who had his sandal loosed from his foot still as respected in Israel after the event as he was before?

The law laid out in Deuteronomy indicates it was originally an act of dishonor to have one's sandal removed in such a manner. In the book of Ruth this method of legalizing transactions appears to have become commonplace. Was it no longer shameful for the kinsman not to stand up to his responsibility?

In our culture, we are often led to believe that what is shameful should be shameless. Christians who believe in moral absolutes are often labeled intolerant, irrelevant or misinformed. It takes courage to stand firm in a society that calls right wrong and looks upon many wrongs as acceptable.

➤ In Philippians 3:8, what value does Paul give to the things he lost in order to gain Christ?

➤ What are some of the costs involved in keeping the nine First Place commitments?

Are you fully willing to do what is right in the sight of God to be able to honor Him? Are you willing to pay the high price it may cost to follow His will? The higher the price you are willing to pay, the more glory He will receive from your service.

Think about the areas in your life in which you might dishonor God. When a weakness comes to mind, confess it to Him. God will give you the strength to overcome it and do what honors Him.

Father God, help me to stand with honor before You as I confess my weaknesses and seek to honor You in all that I do.

Heavenly Father, everything in my life is worth nothing compared to the joy and surpassing greatness of knowing Your Son, Jesus Christ, as Lord and Savior.

DAY 5: *Standing in Prayer*

When the transaction was publicly known in Bethlehem, all the people gathered at the gate and began praying for the future and the family of Ruth and Boaz.

➤ What was the blessing the people asked God to give to Boaz and Ruth (see Ruth 4:11-12)?

➤ What family line was continued with the union of Boaz and Ruth (see Ruth 4:17-22; Matthew 1:1-17)?

➤ Why is the town of Bethlehem of significance?

The greatest family line in the history of humanity was continued through the love between Ruth and Boaz. Could it be that the prayers of the people of the town of Bethlehem made the difference?

Are people praying for you? Do you need to encourage them to keep praying for you? Your strength to honor the Lord comes as a result of prayer. Ask Him to bring to mind those for whom you need to pray. Record their names in your prayer journal or on a page in your Bible study.

➤ What two words are used in James 5:16 to describe a righteous person's prayers?

≫ What did Paul tell Christians to do in 1 Thessalonians 5:16-18?

You can draw constant strength from the Lord through prayer. He desires fellowship with you, not just at mealtime or bedtime, but all the time. You will only be able to stand for Him if you first kneel with Him in prayer.

 Heavenly Father, I come before You on bended knee seeking Your strength to uphold me throughout this day.

Lord, I want to be a prayer warrior for my friends. Help me to always remember the needs of others as I pray each day.

DAY 6: *Reflections*

In this week's study we learned about the promises of God and how to stand firm and with honor in our faith. The memory verse tells us to "let nothing move you. Always give yourselves fully to the work of the Lord."

Standing firm in your faith may sometimes be difficult because of the circumstances around you. Satan will use every opportunity he can to come in and create doubt and conflict in your mind—all the more reason to memorize God's Word. Remember, Paul called God's Word the sword of the Spirit. Scripture is a powerful weapon to use against the nagging whispers of Satan.

Think about various situations in your life where Scripture could be used to help you stand firm in your faith. It may be your health, your job status, conditions at work, serious illness or death in the family, or poor relationships with family members. Anything that drains you of time and energy to be with God becomes a stronghold preventing you from having a closer relationship with God. It is in times like these that the Word of God can be comforting and give you the strength you need to overcome the situation or to go through it with courage.

Build a wall of Scripture against Satan. Let God's Word draw you closer to Him as it separates you from the wiles of Satan. Build it strong, verse by verse. A children's song calls God's love "so wide you can't go around it, so deep you can't go under it, so high you can't go over it." Dear friend, that same love is too wide, too deep and too high for Satan to break through when you are fully ready to seek only God's best for your life.

 Heavenly Father, "I am convinced that neither death nor life, neither angels nor demons, neither the present nor the future, nor any powers, neither height nor depth, nor anything else in all creation, will be able to separate [me] from the love of God that is in Christ Jesus, our Lord" (Romans 8:38-39). Thank You, Father, for that love.

Father God, my present sufferings and difficulties are not worth comparing to the glory that will be revealed in me through Your love and mercy (see Romans 8:18).

Holy Lord, I am fully persuaded that You have the power to do what You have promised, and I stand firm on Your promises (see Romans 4:21).

DAY 7: *Reflections*

As you approach the end of this session in First Place, you can look back and see how much progress you have made from the beginning. Perhaps you spend more time in God's Word through Bible study, or you have found yourself encouraging others in their struggles as they encourage you. If you have been faithful to your commitments and in attendance at meetings, you have grown in your relationship with the Lord. First Place is not a part-time, maybe-I-will, halfhearted attempt at changing a lifestyle. It must be a full-time, yes-I-will, wholehearted effort to seek the best God has for you.

Memorizing the memory verse and other Bible verses gives you a distinct advantage and head start in being victorious over obstacles. Through God's Word you will find strength, prayer, forgiveness, salvation, a way to overcome temptation, rest, a way to defeat sin, a substitute for worry—the list goes on to take care of anything that comes into your life.

Imagine having such an arsenal of weapons ready to battle Satan every day. God is not a part-time, maybe or halfhearted God. He is with you full time with His whole heart. With His Word in your heart and your mind, you are ready to face whatever the day may bring your way. Let His Word become a lamp to your feet and a light for your path (see Psalm 119:105).

The following Scriptures in prayer are examples to use for the things that come into your life and threaten your faith. These verses will help you to stand firm in your faith by standing on the promises of God.

For Strength

O Father, I know I can do everything through You who gives me strength (see Philippians 4:13).

For Forgiveness

Lord, help me to forgive others when they do evil against me just as You, Heavenly Father, have forgiven me. For I know if I cannot forgive others, You will not forgive me (see Matthew 6:14-15).

To Overcome Worry

Holy Lord, Your Word tells me not to worry about food, clothes or my life, for if I first seek Your kingdom and Your righteousness, all these things will be given to me. I will not worry about tomorrow, for tomorrow will worry about itself. Each day has enough trouble of its own (see Matthew 6:33-34).

To Overcome Temptation

Lord God, reach down from on high and take hold of me! Draw me out of deep waters. Rescue me from my powerful enemy, from my foes, who are too strong for me! My enemy has confronted me in the day of my disaster, but You, Lord, are my support! Bring me to a spacious place; rescue me because You delight in me (see Psalm 18:16-19).

To Stand Firm

 Heavenly Father, help me stand firm. Let nothing move me. May I always give myself fully to Your work, O Lord, because I know that my labor in You is not in vain (see 1 Corinthians 15:58).

GROUP PRAYER REQUESTS   TODAY'S DATE:_____

NAME	REQUEST	RESULTS

THE BLESSINGS FROM GOD

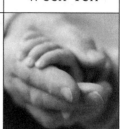

MEMORY VERSE

You prepare a table before me in the presence of my enemies. You anoint my head with oil; my cup overflows. Surely goodness and love will follow me all the days of my life, and I will dwell in the house of the LORD forever.

Psalm 23:5-6

In this week's study, you will discover the ways God blessed the faithful people we have been studying in the book of Ruth. You will also see how God wants to bless all who remain faithful and consistent in their commitment to Him.

DAY 1: *The Blessings of Boaz*

In the book of Ruth, Boaz is a spiritual model for everyone. He honored God by performing his rightful duty as a kinsman-redeemer. He helped those in need when others would not; in fact, he went the second mile to be of service. As a result of his faithfulness, God rewarded him.

➤ According to Ruth 4:13, what are the three blessings Boaz received from the Lord?

To a Jewish family, the conception of a child was as celebrated as the birth. In his culture, Boaz received what only the Lord could give: a wonderful wife and the conception and birth of a child.

➤ According to Ruth 4:17, what was the child's name and who were his son and grandson?

"Obed" means "servant," and it was through Obed's descendants that Jesus, God's own Son, came to serve us (see Matthew 20:28).

Because Boaz obeyed and fulfilled his responsibility, all generations to come would be blessed. Thousands of years later, you seek to serve the One who came to us through this lineage. God's own Son is your blessing today.

After reading Colossians 3:23-25, answer the following:

➤ In whatever we do, what should be our motivation?

➤ What reward is promised to those who serve?

➤ What is promised to those who do wrong?

You will be given a great reward if you are committed to Him and are faithful in your service to Him.

➤ According to Galatians 4:7, what is your reward for your commitment to the Lord?

You are a child of the King. As you go about your responsibilities today, remember the One whom you serve.

 Heavenly Father, thank You for accepting me as a part of Your family, and make me a willing and obedient servant.

Lord Jesus, thank You for the many blessings You have given me when I have put my faith and trust in You.

DAY 2: *The Blessings of Naomi*

Recall the Naomi you met in the first chapter of Ruth. Of all the persons in the story, she suffered the greatest losses and experienced the most bitter of feelings. Yet in the final chapter, she is perhaps the person who felt most blessed.

➢ According to Ruth 4:14-16, what were the rewards Naomi reaped because of her faithfulness?

Naomi's bitterness turned to joy. Her grandchild not only represented security in her old age but the continuation of her husband's lineage. The story of Naomi reminds you not to quit when you are discouraged. Sometimes in your struggle with weight or health or spiritual issues, you will feel as if you are losing the battle. If you stay faithful, as Naomi did, you too can receive blessings. Continue to do the right things in keeping your commitments to First Place.

If you haven't reached your goals in First Place, don't give up. You may get weary in doing the same things over and over, but persevere and keep on doing the commitments and you'll reap your reward.

➢ What is the promise of Galatians 6:9 for those who stick with their goals?

Remember, you will reap your reward if you don't give up. Ask your leader for suggestions for variety in your menus. Try the recipes in the menu plans section of this book or check out the First Place website—www.firstplace.org—for new recipes to try. Continue daily with a prayer and Bible study quiet time with the Lord. Listen to your CD and review your memory verses.

Commit to your exercise program and follow it as carefully as you can. The devil is a master at getting you to quit just before the victory. God will give you encouragement as you seek to achieve goals.

Heavenly Father, give me the stamina I need to keep to my commitments. I don't want to quit before I reach my goals.

Thank You, Father God, for loving me and encouraging me not to grow weary.

DAY 3: *The Blessings of Ruth*

To understand the magnitude of blessings God bestowed on Ruth, you must remember where she started. As a young woman, she experienced the death of her husband before she was able to bear him a child. She then left her own biological family to go to a foreign land to meet a new family. She undoubtedly suffered rejection from some because she was a Gentile in the land of the Jews. She was poor—not much more than a beggar. Her only hope for survival was to be a second-class gleaner.

➤ After reading Ruth 4:13-17 again, list Ruth's blessings.

➤ Who was Ruth's great-grandson?

Ruth had the honor of becoming the great-grandmother of the greatest king ever to rule in Israel. She and Boaz continued the lineage from which the Messiah, Jesus Christ, was born. Aren't we thankful that she didn't stay in Moab?!

➤ What are the names mentioned in Matthew 1:5-6?

The Gentile Ruth is included in the genealogy of Christ! Jesus' roots were not from the rich and famous in the eyes of the world. They were from humble and even sinful folk. Through an impoverished second-class gleaner, a Gentile, an outcast, the Messiah was born. You too were born into a sinful world and you were an outsider, apart from God. You come to Him as a beggar with nothing to commend you, but He made you His child, an heir of God and joint heir with Christ.

Praise God and let Him know how thankful you are for His precious grace. You can be an inspiration and touch people of your generation as Ruth touched hers—and ours.

 Father God, help me to be an example of Your love and grace so that others might be touched by my commitment to You.

Thank You, Lord, for giving us a model such as Ruth, who can show us the way to be obedient to You.

DAY 4: *The Blessings of Israel*

When you are faithfully committed to the work of the Lord, the blessings you receive are often shared with those around you. In this case, the blessings received by Boaz, Naomi and Ruth were shared by the entire nation of Israel.

➛ After reading 1 Samuel 16:1-13, summarize how David came to be chosen as king.

Do you see the significance of the faithfulness of the dear people of Bethlehem during the time of Ruth? Through their lives of faith, God brought Israel their greatest king: David—a man after God's own heart. Surely David's great-grandparents never imagined the glory Israel would receive through them!

➛ Consider your own ancestors; has one of them been an influence in your life?

≫ Have you carried on a tradition or family custom in your own life? Describe it.

You have a responsibility to the family of God to carry on the blessings you have received and share them with others.

≫ What are some of the blessings you have received as a child of God?

≫ Read Romans 8:18; then write the verse in your own words.

Look past the pain of any suffering you may be enduring right now. God will bring glory through the suffering.

≫ Think back to a time when God turned troublesome circumstances into a blessing. Briefly describe it.

 Heavenly Father, thank You for seeing me through the troublesome times in my life and for giving me blessings.

Thank You, Father God, that nothing can separate me from Your love in Christ Jesus.

DAY 5: *The Blessings for You*

You are blessed by the miraculous way God formed the Messiah's family. You are also blessed by knowing that God has a divine plan for your life, just as He had for the persons you've been studying.

➤ What are some of the words and phrases found in Psalm 23 that remind you of God's daily presence in your life?

➤ Write your memory verse from this passage—from memory.

Did you think about the fact that these words were penned by Boaz and Ruth's great-grandson? Surely he had heard the family stories of their courtship and marriage, which may have encouraged his faith in God. David was convinced that God is the One who leads you down your life's path.

Another way you are blessed is through Jesus Himself. Not only did He die to save you from your sin, but He also lives today at God's side to intercede on your behalf.

➤ What is the promise in Hebrews 7:25?

Without a doubt, Jesus has had your best in mind from before the beginning of the world. Read Matthew 6:33, the First Place theme verse (or recite it from memory!).

➤ What can you expect when you seek Christ's kingdom above all else?

Ruth and Naomi could not have dreamed how their commitment to God would change the world. How has keeping the nine commitments of First Place changed your world? What changes are yet to come? You may want to consider each commitment separately in your prayer journal.

You seek God's best because He desires to give you His best! Jesus said, "Ask and it will be given to you" (Matthew 7:7). Let this study of the book of Ruth encourage you to believe that God wants only His best for you. Thank Him for His great love and grace that makes living an abundant life possible.

Thank You, Father God, for being my shepherd and guiding me through each day of my life.

Dear Lord, thank You for Your great love for me and Your grace that enables me to live a more abundant life.

DAY 6: *Reflections*

Your memory verse for this week comes from one of the best-known passages in the Bible. This psalm is one many people memorize in its entirety. It is often repeated by those in need, in pain or facing death. This psalm is a perfect example of how memorized Scripture comes to mind in times when comfort is needed.

If memorizing Scripture is a problem for you, begin with verses with which you are familiar, such as the Twenty-third Psalm. Beginning with the familiar gives you an edge as you already know the words. Many times the most difficult part is remembering where a Scripture is found. Repeating the source, or reference, at both the beginning and the end will help you glue it to the verse.

Three reasons to memorize Scripture can be found in this psalm. First, memorized Scripture can be used in handling difficult situations—"Even though I walk through the valley of the shadow of death, I will fear no evil, for you are with me" (v. 4). Second, it can be used to overcome temptation—"The LORD is my shepherd, I shall not be in want" (v. 1). Third, it gives guidance—"He guides me in the paths of righteousness" (v. 3).

Knowledge of the Scriptures and the strength that comes when you are able to quote them is an important part of putting on the full armor of God. Focus on your memory verse for each week. Repeat it every morning and every evening and at various times during the day. God will honor your efforts.

Heavenly Father, I know the grass withers and the flowers fade away, but Your love endures forever (see Isaiah 40:8).

Holy God, thank You for Your promise that when I go through fire or through water, You will bring me out to great enrichment (see Isaiah 43:2).

Father, You have promised that if I call upon You, You will answer me. You will be with me in time of trouble, and You will deliver me and give me honor (see Psalm 91:15).

DAY 7: *Reflections*

As you come to the end of this session in First Place, our prayer for you is that you will not count your success or failure in terms of how many pounds you lost. Your leaders are more interested in your spiritual victories than your physical ones, although your weight loss is a concern as well.

What are your spiritual victories? Memorizing your weekly memory verses, being able to follow the commitments week to week and establishing a daily quiet time with God in prayer and Bible study can be victories for you. If you didn't meet all your goals, don't give up. God isn't finished with you yet. He wants you to continue with the lifestyle you find in First Place.

Look back over the memory verses for each week. Think about how each can be used as you seek God's best for you. Put on the whole armor of God and go forth into the world. Armed with the sword of the Spirit, you will be able to conquer your foes.

Make the First Place lifestyle your lifestyle whether you are in a First Place group or not. Continue with your daily Bible studies, Scripture memory, prayer, exercise and Live-It plan. God will lead you to victory.

If possible, obtain a copy of Beth Moore's book *Praying God's Word*. Use it as a tool to help you memorize Scripture and use Scripture in your prayers. Beth addresses all the strongholds, or obstacles, that threaten to come in and keep you from having an intimate relationship with God.

Lord God, help me not to be overcome by evil but to overcome evil with good (see Romans 12:21).[1]

Blessed am I because my transgressions are forgiven.

Blessed am I because my sins are covered. May my deep gratitude be evident in the way I relate to others (see Psalm 32:1).[2]

I humble myself, therefore, under Your mighty hand, God, that You may lift me up in due time. I cast all this anxiety on You because You care for me (see 1 Peter 5:6-7).[3]

You have shown me what is good. And what do You, Lord, require of me? To act justly and to love mercy and to walk humbly with my God (see Micah 6:8).[4]

Heavenly Father, "You [have prepared] a table before me in the presence of my enemies. You anoint my head with oil; my cup overflows. Surely goodness and love will follow me all the days of my life, and I will dwell in the house of the LORD forever" (Psalm 23:5-6).

Notes
1. Beth Moore, *Praying God's Word* (Nashville, TN: Broadman and Holman, 2000), p. 228.
2. Ibid.
3. Ibid., p. 231.
4. Ibid.

GROUP PRAYER REQUESTS TODAY'S DATE:_____

NAME	REQUEST	RESULTS

DIETARY SUPPLEMENTS—

MIRACLE OR MYTH?

It seems like every time you turn around there's new information about vitamins, minerals and other supplements. If you're like most people, you may be confused about what to do! What's true and what isn't?

HEADLINES—SORTING THROUGH THE HYPE

- There are no miracle foods or supplements. Avoid anything that promises rapid results or a quick fix.
- Ignore dramatic statements that go against what most physicians, registered dietitians or national health organizations are saying.
- Stick to what you know about good nutrition, regular physical activity and a healthy lifestyle. Eating a well-balanced diet that includes a wide variety of foods is the best way to obtain the nutrients you need.
- Your best bet is to avoid anything that sounds too good to be true!

It's true—vitamins, minerals and phytochemicals are necessary for good health and provide many great benefits! However, the true benefit comes from food, not from supplements.

> Then God said, "I give you every seed-bearing plant on the face of the whole earth and every tree that has fruit with seed in it. They will be yours for food" (Genesis 1:29).

While we all know it's important to eat fruits and vegetables, only 20 percent of adults meet the minimum recommendation of five servings of fruits and vegetables each day. How many servings do you eat? Never substitute other foods in your Live-It plan for the fruits, vegetables and whole grains that you need to eat. Better yet, get lots of regular physical activity and add in a few extra servings. You've probably heard that more is not necessarily better. When it comes to fruits and vegetables, studies show that eating seven or more servings may offer additional health benefits.

VITAMINS AND MINERALS—ENERGY IN A PILL!

Not likely. Vitamins and minerals do not supply energy—that's the job of calories from carbohydrates and fats. However, vitamins and minerals are a part of the process of changing the food you eat into energy your body can use. They're also important for many chemical reactions that take place in your body every day. The best scientific evidence suggests that your body uses vitamins and minerals best in the combinations found naturally in food.

HEADLINES! HEADLINES! READ ALL ABOUT IT!

It seems like new information about vitamins makes the news every month. You may have heard about antioxidants, homocysteine and phytochemicals. The following are brief explanations of what medical science has discovered:

- **Antioxidants**—Three antioxidants are most often in the headlines: beta carotene, vitamin E and vitamin C. Antioxidants help maintain healthy cells by protecting them against oxidation and the damaging effects of free radicals. Free radicals are potentially damaging oxygen molecules that are produced naturally by the body. Some experts believe that environmental factors such as smoking, air pollution and other stressors increase the production of free radicals. Studies suggest that antioxidants in fruits, vegetables and other foods may help reduce the risk of heart disease, certain cancers and a variety of other health problems. Most experts feel that more studies need to be done before specific recommendations for supplementation can be made.

- **Homocysteine**—You may have heard about homocysteine—a protein in the blood. High levels may be associated with an increased risk of heart attack and stroke. Homocysteine levels can be influenced by what you eat. The B vitamins—folic acid, B_6 and B_{12}—help to break down homocysteine in the body. So far, there are no studies showing that taking B vitamins will lower your risk for heart attack and stroke. Everyone should follow an eating plan that has plenty of folic acid and vitamins B_6 and B_{12}. Good sources of these are citrus fruits, tomatoes, dark-green leafy vegetables and fortified cereals and grain products (rice, oats and wheat flour). Eggs, fish, chicken and lean red meats are also good sources.

- **Phytochemicals**—Phytochemicals—plant chemicals—are substances that plants naturally produce to protect themselves against disease. These same compounds appear to have very beneficial effects on our health as well. You may have heard about some of these: isoflavones, sulphoranes, lycopene and other carotenoids to name a few. At this time, there is no evidence that these chemicals can be concentrated in pill form to provide health benefits. Take your phytochemicals in the form of fruits, vegetables and whole grains.

Questions and Answers

Do I Need to Take Supplements?

Currently none of the major health organizations such as the American Heart Association, the American Cancer Society or the American Dietetic Association recommend that healthy adults routinely take vitamin or mineral supplements for general health. There's simply not enough information on the dosages or combinations of vitamins, minerals and other nutrients that work best—or work at all!

For the time being, it is best to get the more than 100 vitamins, minerals and phytochemicals your body needs from the foods you eat. Supplements simply cannot recreate what God has done naturally with fruits, vegetables, whole grains and other nutritious foods. Eat a variety of fruits, vegetables and whole grains each day. Balance these foods with lean meats and low-fat dairy products to get the balance and variety you need for a vitamin-packed eating plan.

What If I'm Already Taking Vitamin and Mineral Supplements?

There is no evidence that taking a multivitamin and mineral supplement that does not exceed the Recommended Daily Allowances (RDAs) is associated with any harmful effects. Vitamin and mineral supplements can be an important part of an overall health plan if taking them helps you to live a healthier lifestyle—i.e., eating a healthy diet and being more physically active. However, dietary supplements are not a substitute for eating healthy! Vitamin and mineral doses higher than the RDAs should only be taken after seeking advice from your physician or a registered dietitian. For otherwise healthy people, there is only limited data suggesting advantages for taking certain vitamin or mineral supplements in excess of the RDAs.

Are Dietary Supplements More Appropriate for Some People?

Supplements may be appropriate for some people.

- Osteoporosis, iron deficiency, digestive disorders and other health conditions may be treated or prevented with certain dietary supplements.
- People who follow very low-calorie eating plans or restrictive eating patterns (such as a vegetarian who consumes no meat or dairy foods) may need supplements. However, we do not recommend these restrictive eating plans.
- People who can't eat certain foods may need a supplement to give the body what it needs.
- Women planning to become pregnant or who are pregnant/breast feeding should talk to their doctor about the need for certain supplements such as folic acid and iron.

Whatever you do, work at it with all your heart, as working for the Lord,
not for men, since you know that you will receive an
inheritance from the Lord as a reward.
Colossians 3:23-24

Work is a necessary part of life. It can provide both joy and satisfaction. Unfortunately, it also brings schedules, deadlines, long hours and many other responsibilities and stresses. The fast pace of work life often makes it hard to make healthy choices on the job. Pressures and responsibilities at work are common reasons people give for not taking better care of themselves.

You have to make taking care of yourself a priority while on the job. Prayerfully consider ways to make healthy living a part of your workday. Ask family, friends and coworkers to help you find creative ways to do what you need to do. You can generally find several minutes during the day to do something good for yourself. Look at your typical workday: Are you eating healthy? Do you make time for physical activity? How do you deal with job-related stress?

Here are some suggestions and tips to help you get started. Don't try to change everything at once. Start with those changes you're most ready to make and most confident you can change.

EAT HEALTHY

- Never skip meals. Your body needs food throughout the day for energy. Start your day with a nutritious breakfast and don't skip lunch. Every meal you miss robs your body of important nutrients. Also, skipping meals will make it more likely that you'll overeat later.
- Prepare and take your own food—brown-bag it! You're much more likely to eat healthy meals and snacks if you prepare them yourself. The key is planning ahead.

1. Healthy eating at work begins at the grocery store. Make a list of foods you enjoy and that are easy for you to bring to work. Choose fresh, canned or dried fruits, raw or canned vegetables, lean sandwich meats, low-fat crackers, bean or broth-based soups, low-fat milk and yogurt.
2. Cook extra portions with evening meals and pack the leftovers for work—homemade fast food.
3. If you don't have a refrigerator at work, bring an ice cooler or insulated lunch bag. Buy plastic containers in which you can store foods and beverages.
4. Store healthy snacks in your desk drawer, briefcase or car. Low-fat crackers, graham crackers, cookies, bagels, fresh or dried fruit, cereal, popcorn and instant oatmeal are all great choices.

🍎 If you eat out, choose your restaurants and your meals carefully.

1. Watch your portion sizes; they are usually much more than you need.
2. Split your meal with a companion or box some up and bring it home.
3. Avoid fried foods and dishes cooked with heavy sauces or lots of cheese. Choose bean or broth-based soups, baked or grilled chicken, fresh salads with a low-fat dressing, steamed vegetables, sandwiches with lean meat and fresh fruit.
4. Find two or three restaurants where you know you can make healthy choices; recommend these when eating out.

BE MORE PHYSICALLY ACTIVE

Fit physical activity into your workday whenever you can. Even 5 to 10 minutes of activity done throughout the day can improve your health and fitness.

🍎 Schedule activity into your day just like you do important meetings.

🍎 Park your car further away from your office building.

🍎 Take the stairs instead of the elevator. Use the bathroom on at least the next floor up or across the building.

- Hand deliver messages rather than use office mail, the computer or telephone.
- Take 10- to 15-minute walking breaks.
- Stand up and do some stretching while you're talking on the phone.
- Buy some handheld weights or elastic exercise bands to use in your office.
- Go for a walk during your lunch hour.
- Start a walking group or aerobic dance class at work.
- Make time for physical activity when you travel—walk in the airport between flights.
- Suggest that your company purchase a few pieces of exercise equipment.

REDUCE STRESS

You may not be able to eliminate the stress of your job, but you can learn to handle it in more positive ways. Here are some tips to help you reduce and respond more positively to stress you may experience on the job. Stress often begins before you arrive: running late, responsibilities at home and fighting traffic.

- Get organized before you leave for work. It's best to do most of your preparation the night before.
- Be sure to get enough sleep. Most people need seven to nine hours of sleep every night. Discover how much sleep you need and try to get it every night.
- Arrange your schedule so that you can avoid driving in heavy traffic.
- Leave your home early enough so that you're not rushed.
- Take time to relax before you leave for work or while you're in the car: breathe deeply, relax your muscles, pray or listen to relaxing music or the Bible on tape. This is also a great time to listen to your First Place Memory Verses CD.
- At work, once or twice a day take 10 or 15 minutes to relax and organize the rest of your day.

- Prioritize your daily and weekly activities.
- Learn to recognize things that are less important or not important at all.
- Schedule time for yourself.
- Focus on one thing at a time.
- Learn to say "No!" or "I need help!"
- Personalize your workspace with pictures and special messages.
- Avoid cigarette smoke and limit caffeine intake.
- Friends and family can offer encouragement and support during stressful times. Look for ways to share responsibilities with others. Think of specific things people can do to help you reduce your stress.
- Set aside time each week to discuss issues, plans, schedules and responsibilities with your family, friends and coworkers. Make this a time for teamwork and positive problem solving.
- Make time to enjoy yourself outside of work. You need to get away and take time for yourself and loved ones.

➤ What are some things you're ready to do to lower stress on the job?

HOME FITNESS EQUIPMENT

Do you just not have time to make it to the fitness center? Do you feel uncomfortable working out in front of others? Maybe you don't have a fitness center nearby. Is a fitness center membership more than you're willing or able to pay? Maybe you would just like to have a backup for those days when you can't make it to the gym? Fortunately, you don't have to join a fitness center to get the benefits of physical activity. There are many great ways to fit physical activity into your life. Choose activities that you enjoy and can fit into your lifestyle. With a little planning, you can get all the physical activity you need in the comfort and convenience of your own home.

THE ADVANTAGES OF HOME EXERCISE

- Convenience—no travel time and no special hours are required, and you don't have to worry about what to wear.
- Privacy—you can work out in the comfort of your own home and at your own speed with no overcrowding.
- Cost—depending on what activity and equipment you choose, exercising at home can be very economical.

THE DISADVANTAGES OF HOME EXERCISE

- Less variety—a fitness center offers a greater variety of exercise and equipment options.
- Self-discipline—some people have a hard time motivating themselves to work out alone.
- Distractions—the television, telephone, spouse, kids and household chores may compete for your time and attention.
- Cost—some fitness equipment may cost as much or more than a club membership.

Types of Equipment

There is no best exercise or piece of exercise equipment. The best one is the one that is right for you. Any activity that requires you to use your muscles or causes you to breathe a little harder is good for your body. Walking, jogging, bicycling, dancing and strength training are good examples. Choose the one you like best and do it regularly.

All of the following types of exercise equipment are good choices:

- Treadmills
- Skiing machines
- Elastic exercise bands
- Stationary or regular bicycles
- Rowers
- Stair climbers
- Strength equipment
- Jump ropes
- Aerobic or step videos
- Roller blades or skates

Don't just buy a piece of exercise equipment because you think it will be good for you. Consider what types of activity you enjoy. Ask yourself these important questions before you buy:

- *What do I enjoy doing?*
- *Will I really enjoy working out at home? Why?*
- *Will I use the equipment regularly? Will I quickly get bored with it?* Far too common is the exercise machine that becomes an expensive clothes rack or ends up in a garage sale or thrift shop!
- *Have I used or bought home-exercise equipment before? What did I like about it? What did I dislike about it?*
- *Do I have a convenient and comfortable place to put it?*
- *How much can I afford to spend?* Set a budget before you go shopping.

Selection Tips

When shopping for exercise equipment, look for something that gives you the feel of the activity you enjoy. You need to test equipment before you buy it. Does it seem to be well made? Does it feel solid and durable? Give the equipment a good test ride—five minutes is not enough!

Stationary Bike

Stationary bikes can provide a great low impact workout and don't take up much space.

- Choose a bike with a smooth pedaling motion.
- Make sure you're comfortable with the pedaling resistance and that it's easily adjusted.
- A comfortable, adjustable-tilt seat is a must. If bicycle seats are typically uncomfortable for you, look for a recumbent bike which allows you to sit in a padded chair with your legs extended in front of you.
- Some bikes have arm levers that allow you to work your upper body too.

Treadmill

If you enjoy walking or jogging, a treadmill may be right for you.

- You'll need plenty of room—both in length and width—to comfortably walk or jog.
- The walking or jogging surface should be stable and provide good shock absorption (i.e., doesn't bounce or rock back and forth).
- Choose a machine with handrails for balance and a control panel that is easy to reach and use. It's best if you can adjust the speed and elevation while exercising.
- Strong motors (1.25 to 1.75 horsepower) make for a quieter and longer-lasting treadmill.

Stair-Climbing Machine

A stair-climbing machine gives you a good low-impact workout in a small space.

- Choose a sturdy machine with good stability.
- Look for independent steps that have a smooth motion; chain or cable systems are generally smoother than hydraulic (air-powered) systems.

- It should allow for variable resistance (i.e., you set the tension, or workload).
- Make sure it is equipped with comfortable handrails.

Cross-Country Skiing and Rowing Machines

- Look for a machine that works both the upper and lower body.
- Look for stability; the machine shouldn't rock back and forth.
- The machine should provide smooth sliding motion of skis, seat and arm pulleys.
- Make sure it allows for variable resistance (i.e., you set the tension, or workload).

Weights

Weights are good for increasing strength and bone density.

- Multistation resistance machines certainly have their place, but they are not affordable or practical for everyone.
- You can get all the strength training you need with handheld weights, elastic exercise bands, dumbbells and an exercise mat or bench.

ADDITIONAL TIPS

- If you know someone with home exercise equipment, ask to try it out before buying your own.
- Analyze your workout room. The area you plan to exercise in should be spacious and pleasant with good lighting and ventilation. Some people like to read or watch television while using their exercise equipment.
- Because you must test the equipment extensively before you purchase it; wear your workout gear when shopping!
- Buy from a knowledgeable retailer. Discuss warranties, installation, maintenance and service plans.
- Check out used equipment for purchase.

MANAGING YOUR TIME

Time—there never seems to be enough of it. Yet God has given each one of us all the time we need: 60 minutes in an hour, 24 hours in a day and 168 hours in a week. Getting everything done within these time limits is quite a challenge. Obligations at home, work and church compete with less-important activities for your time. The key is focusing on the important activities and eliminating those that are not important. Some things should take priority: spending time with the Lord, taking care of yourself and serving others. Are you making time for worship, prayer, Bible study, communication with family and friends, rest, healthy nutrition, regular physical activity and work? Gaining control of your time helps you move through life with peace and purpose.

A TIME TO CHANGE

Time—or lack of it—is one of the most common barriers Americans cite for not eating well. What's the number one excuse for not exercising regularly? You guessed it—lack of time! Convenience is one of the most important factors people consider when selecting a meal or including exercise in their day.

It's true that lifestyle change takes time. Achieving and maintaining a healthy weight by following the First Place commitments will take time. Unfortunately, there are no extra hours in a day. Trying to keep pace with all you have to do can be frustrating and stressful. By simplifying your life and organizing your time you can improve your health and quality of life.

PERSONAL TIME INVENTORY

The first step in managing your time is to know how you spend it. Use the following inventory to find out where and how you spend your time.

First, during the next several days evaluate how much time you actually spend in the following activities; use the extra spaces to fill in activities not on the list. Write in the hours you spend in each activity daily or weekly; choose what works best for you. Try to account for as much of the 24 hours in a day or the 168 hours in a week as possible.

Next, use the inventory to determine the ideal amount of time you would like to spend in each activity.

Actual Time I Spend on Activities

Activity	Hrs.	Activity	Hrs.	Activity	Hrs.
Bible study		Grooming		Recreation	
Church		Housework		Shopping	
Cooking/dining		Paying bills		Sleeping	
Daydreaming		Physical activity		Social activities	
Driving/travel		Prayer		Telephone	
Family time		Reading		Television	
Working					

Ideal Time I Would Like to Spend on Activities

Activity	Hrs.	Activity	Hrs.	Activity	Hrs.
Bible study		Grooming		Recreation	
Church		Housework		Shopping	
Cooking/dining		Paying bills		Sleeping	
Daydreaming		Physical activity		Social activities	
Driving/travel		Prayer		Telephone	
Family time		Reading		Television	
Working					

After completing your Personal Time Inventory, review how much time you spend in each activity. Compare this with your inventory of how much time you would ideally like to spend on each activity. See what activities are taking up too much of your time. Prayerfully ask God to help you learn where and how to make better use of your time.

Making a plan to plan is the most important step in using your time wisely. Set aside time each day to review your plans for the day and upcoming week. What is the best time of day for you? Is it in the morning? Or maybe at night? You also need to set aside several hours each month, or at least every three months, to review where you've been, what you've done and where you are going. Look at both your short- and long-term goals. What changes do you need to make? What projects have you completed and what goals have you achieved?

TIME-SAVING TIPS

- Keep a calendar or daily organizer to keep track of all your appointments and plans. Write everything down and review it often.
- Learn to use a checklist to keep track of your day's events. Use your organizer and checklist to help you get into a routine.
- Always give yourself time to review your goals, responsibilities and schedule before adding new things. Learn to say no to things that aren't a good use of your time.
- Stick with one or two important tasks each day. Keep a wish list of things you need to do or would like to do once you finish the important tasks.
- When making your daily, weekly and long-term plans, make sure you schedule time to take care of yourself: physical activity, relaxation and fun times with family and friends.
- Don't expect everything to go perfectly; just do the best you can.
- Do the difficult things first! Try not to put off too much until tomorrow.
- Break big projects into smaller pieces. Reward yourself for completing each step.
- Learn to ask family and friends for the help you need.
- Make a list of the activities with which you need help; be specific.
- Make a list of specific people who can help you with each activity.
- Determine who can help with household chores: taking out the trash, doing dishes, mowing the grass, running errands.
- Who can help you at work? What can they do?
- Have someone hold you accountable for organizing your time. Ask them to review with you how you spend your time. Ask them to help you eliminate those activities that are less important.

A PLAN TO CHANGE

➣ What are the top three reasons you don't use your time as wisely as you would like: lack of organization, letting others control your time, too many responsibilities, wasting time, procrastination? List your reasons here. Be specific!

1.

2.

3.

Next, determine three steps you can take to overcome each of these time wasters. List the steps here. Start with the area you're most ready and confident you can change. Work through each step, trying to make each one a habit before moving on to the next.

Reason One	Reason Two	Reason Three

UNDERSTANDING FAD DIETS

Lose Weight Without Exercising!
Take Off Pounds While You Sleep!
Lose 30 Pounds in 30 Days!
Zap 3 Inches from Your Thighs!

Does it seem like everywhere you turn there's a new miracle diet or supplement being advertised or reported in the media? Sometimes all the headlines can be overwhelming. In fact, one of the biggest reasons people give for not starting or sticking with a healthy eating plan is confusion and frustration over all the conflicting information. Do you ever wonder how you can ever separate the fact from the fiction?

It is estimated that Americans spend over $30 billion each year on products and plans to lose weight. Despite all the money people spend, only 5 percent are successful in losing weight over the long term. Look back over your dieting history.

YOUR DIETING HISTORY

➤ Have you ever tried a diet or supplement that promised more than it could deliver?

☐ Yes ☐ No

➤ If you answered yes, what diets or products have you tried?

➤ Why didn't these programs or products work for you?

It's important to realize that no diet, pill or product can produce the benefits that come with following God's plan for healthy living. You are truly "fearfully and wonderfully made" (Psalm 139:14). The secret to good health and effective living is deciding to care for your body as God's good creation (see 1 Corinthians 6:19-20). Are you ready to commit to a healthy lifestyle of good nutrition and regular physical activity?

PLAN EVALUATION

Remember, no food, diet or product provides all the magic answers for good health or weight loss. To help you sort through the confusion, use the following checklist when evaluating information:

- ☐ Does the program promise a quick fix?
- ☐ Do the claims sound too good to be true; are the words "breakthrough" or "miracle" used to describe it?
- ☐ Does the program recommend regular physical activity?
- ☐ Are only certain foods or products emphasized? Are other foods off-limits?
- ☐ Do you have to buy special supplements or products?
- ☐ Can you follow the program for a lifetime?
- ☐ Does the program go against the recommendation of major nutrition, medical and scientific organizations?

THE FACTS ABOUT FAD DIETS

Most fad diets are recycled every few years with a few new twists added to make them seem different. The following are some common fad diets and things to look out for:

1. Many fad diets take advantage of people's desire for instant results by creating the myth that certain foods or supplements have special physiologic or metabolic properties for quick weight loss. There are no known miracle foods or supplements that burn fat or promote long-term weight loss.

A weight loss of one to two pounds per week is all that the body can healthfully lose. More rapid weight loss is the result of water loss, not fat loss. Over the long term some of these diets will even result in muscle loss—especially if physical activity is not involved.

These diets are usually unbalanced and don't provide the variety you need for good health or enjoyable eating. *A calorie is a calorie,* whether it comes from fat, protein or carbohydrate. You gain weight when you take in more calories than your body needs.

2. Some fad diets suggest that eating foods in certain combinations will help you burn fat more effectively, boost your metabolism or improve your health. These diets, like the ones that promote miracle foods, don't work! God did not design your body in a way that makes eating a complicated affair. Digestion is an amazing process that uses specific enzymes in specific areas of your digestive track. Combinations of certain foods, timing of meals or special supplements do not have any effect on this process. Another problem with these diets is that they don't provide the variety and balance your body needs for good health.

3. Most fad diets don't encourage physical activity. In fact, some programs promise weight loss while you sleep! Physical activity should be one of the highest priorities of any weight-loss program. Few people can maintain long-term weight loss without regular physical activity.

4. Avoid diets that offer a one-size-fits-all approach. There is no one diet that works for everyone. Weight regulation is a complex process that involves many factors. A good weight-loss program—such as First Place—considers each person as an individual. A good program allows you to personalize your eating plan. You are more likely to stick to a plan that most closely reflects your lifestyle, tastes and preferences.

5. Fad diets may offer easy access to over-the-counter weight-loss drugs or supplements. Studies show that even approved weight-loss medications result in a weight loss of only 10 to 15 percent; it's unlikely that a product advertised in the back of a magazine or on the side of the road will be any more effective. Some of these supplements may even cause serious side effects—even death! Never take a medication or supplement without talking to your primary doctor.

6. Many diet programs sell packaged foods. Liquid meal replacements are especially popular. Liquid meal replacements can help increase

weight loss in the short term, but studies show that they are no more effective than other methods in promoting long-term weight loss. These products may make a lot of money for the commercial programs, but they may not be the most effective way to teach people how to develop and follow a healthy eating plan. To be effective, a weight-loss program must teach people how to develop lifelong habits of healthy eating and regular physical activity. This includes learning how to choose and prepare healthy foods.

7. Many programs are sold by self-proclaimed experts. These experts make sensational claims about breakthrough diets, ancient secrets, scientific research and miracle foods or supplements that they have discovered or developed. Often these programs are promoted using personal success stories of famous television, film or sports celebrities. The most reliable spokespersons have training in nutrition and medicine from reputable universities. Contact groups such as the American Dietetics Association, the American Heart Association and the American Medical Society to see if the program or product is supported by major nutrition, medical and scientific organizations. Registered dietitians (RDs) are also a good source of nutrition information.

UNDERSTANDING METABOLISM

The process by which your body transforms calories from the foods you eat into energy is called metabolism. Metabolism is a complex process that is regulated by your nervous system, hormones, age, body composition and physical activity. Heredity may also influence metabolism. Every person has a unique metabolism; unfortunately, some bodies run slower than others!

METABOLIC RATES

Your body is constantly using energy, or burning calories—even at rest! In fact, most of the energy or calories your body uses every day just keep it running: heart beating, lungs breathing, brain thinking, etc. Your *resting metabolic rate*—what doctors call your BMR—is responsible for burning approximately 60 to 70 percent of your daily calories.

Calculating Your Resting Metabolic Rate

Men 66 + (6.2 x _____ weight in pounds)	+ (12.7 x _____ height in inches)	− (6.8 x age)	
Women 655 + (4.4 x _____ weight in pounds)	+ (4.3 x _____ height in inches)	− (4.7 x age)	
(_____) +	(_____) +	(_____)	− (_____)
		=	_____

THE IMPORTANCE OF BODY COMPOSITION

Body composition—how much muscle and fat you have—determines a large part of your resting metabolism. A lean and fit body has a higher metabolism than one that's overweight and out of shape. Women tend to have slightly slower metabolic rates than men primarily because they have less muscle. With aging and inactivity, muscle mass goes down, body fat goes up and metabolism slows down. Weight goes up, too, if eating habits don't change. Body weight also affects metabolism. Believe it or not, studies show that overweight people generally have higher metabolisms than their normal-weight counterparts.

To be in energy—or weight—balance you must burn as many calories in daily living as you take in from the foods you eat. Regardless of whether your metabolism is fast or slow, the system works the same for everyone and the formula to lose weight is the same for everyone: *Eat less and exercise more!*

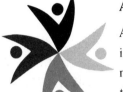

A Calorie Is a Calorie

A calorie is a measure of energy much as an inch is a measure of distance and a pound is a measure of weight. Calories are stored in three important nutrients: fats, protein and carbohydrates. While fat contains more than twice the calories of proteins or carbohydrates, it doesn't have any special fattening properties. *When your body takes in more calories than it needs, the excess calories are stored as body fat whether the calories come from fat, protein or carbohydrate.* In fact, many studies show that low-fat eating plans are no more effective at reducing body fat than other plans.

The Fitness and Activity Advantage

Fortunately, with a little effort you can increase your metabolism and change your body composition. Actually, physical activity accounts for 15 to 30 percent of your daily energy expenditure. Even moderate physical activities such as brisk walking, bicycling or swimming can burn *an extra 300 to 400 calories per hour.* Add in other daily activities such as taking the stairs, walking the dog and working in the yard, and you've become a calorie-burning machine! Physical activity also helps by allowing you to maintain and even build muscle.

Estimating Your Daily Calorie Needs

Multiply your resting metabolic rate _____ x	1.2 if you're sedentary* 1.4 if you're moderately active** 1.6 if you're vigorously active***	= _____

*Sedentary = normal daily activities only.
**Moderate = ≥ 30 min of activities such as brisk walking at least 3 days a week.
***Vigorous = activities such as running at least 5 days a week.

How does this calorie level compare to the calorie level you chose on the "Choosing a Calorie Level" worksheet from the *First Place Member's Guide?* How does it compare to the calorie level you're currently following for your Live-it Plan? It's probably a little higher, because we subtracted a few calories to allow for weight loss.

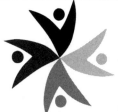 Since it takes approximately 3,500 calories to burn a pound of fat, changing your calorie balance by 500 calories each day will result in a weight loss of one pound each week (1,000 calories equals two pounds). You can change your energy balance by cutting back on calories or increasing physical activity: *It's best to do both!*

Putting It All Together

The above calculations are only estimates; however, they allow you to get a reasonable idea of how many calories your body needs each day. By monitoring your weight over time, you can fine-tune this estimate to get an idea of your body's metabolism. Unfortunately, some people do have slower metabolisms. If this applies to you, you'll need to gradually cut back on calories and increase your physical activity until you see the scale show that you're losing an average of one to two pounds each week or approximately five pounds each month. You may need to change your calorie level as you go. Reevaluate your plan every one to two months based on how well you are reaching your goals. Use your CR (Commitment Record) and your Personal Weight Record to help you keep track.

THE DOWNSIDE OF DIETING

Studies show that the body adapts to dieting and weight loss by slowing down its metabolism. One reason this happens is that dieting and weight loss result in some muscle loss. This slowdown is also a natural response to a lower body weight and may serve to protect the body against extreme calorie restriction. Unfortunately, this makes it more difficult to maintain long-term weight loss. It's important to realize that after you lose weight, your body will need *fewer* calories than *before* you lost weight. Some experts believe that yo-yo dieting—the process of using an extreme diet to lose weight quickly and then gaining back what you've lost (and then some) when you stop dieting and resume your original eating habits—also slows the metabolic rate over time. This may happen because with each weight-loss attempt, the body loses muscle mass. When the body gains the weight back, much of it is body fat. The good news is that as you become more physically active, you will be able to eat a few more calories and still maintain your weight.

THE WEIGHT LOSS PLATEAU

Most people will experience periods when weight loss seems to stop; we call this a plateau. Your body hits a plateau because as weight drops, it requires fewer calories to keep it running. When this happens, be patient. Give your body time to adjust to its new weight. Increasing the frequency, intensity or duration of your activity may help you get through this period, but be careful not to increase your activity too fast! You can also adjust your calorie intake downward, but be careful not to go too low; women should never go below 1200 calories, and men should not go below 1500 calories.

 Believe it or not, another 5 to 10 percent of your metabolism goes into digesting the foods you eat. This process is called the thermogenesis of food. Some fad diets use this physiological principle to mislead dieters into following programs that rely on meal timing and special food combinations. The effects of the thermogenesis of food on daily energy expenditure are small at best and no foods have the ability to burn fat.

FIRST PLACE
MENU PLANS

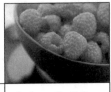

Each plan is based on approximately 1400 calories.

Breakfast	2 breads, 1 fruit, 1 milk, 0-½ fat (When a meat exchange is used, milk is omitted.)
Lunch	2 meats, 2 breads, 1 vegetable, 1 fruit, 1 fat
Dinner	3 meats, 2 breads, 2 vegetables, 1 fat
Snacks	1 bread, 1 fruit, 1 milk, ½-1 fat (or any remaining exchanges)

For more calories, add the following to the 1400 calorie plan.

1600 calories	2 breads, 1 fat
1800 calories	2 meats, 3 breads, 1 vegetable, 1 fat
2000 calories	2 meats, 4 breads, 1 vegetable, 3 fats
2200 calories	2 meats, 5 breads, 1 vegetable, 1 fruit, 5 fats
2400 calories	2 meats, 6 breads, 2 vegetables, 1 fruit, 6 fats

The exchanges for these meals were calculated using the MasterCook software. It uses a database of over 6,000 food items prepared using United States Department of Agriculture (USDA) publications and information from food manufacturers. As with any nutritional program, MasterCook calculates the nutritional values of the recipes based on ingredients. Nutrition may vary due to how the food is prepared, where the food comes from, i.e., geography, soil content, season, ripeness, processing and method of preparation. For these reasons, please use the recipes and menu plans as approximate guides. As always consult your physician and/or a registered dietician before starting a diet program.

Menu Plans for Two Weeks

🍎 Breakfasts

1 slice diet multigrain bread
1 tsp. all-fruit spread
1 c. nonfat plain yogurt topped with
2 tbsp. Grape Nuts
½ c. blueberries
Exchanges: 2 breads, 1 fruit, 1 milk, ½ fat

~~~~~~

1 English muffin
1 egg, poached
½ grapefruit
Exchanges: 1 meat, 2 breads, 1 fruit, ½ fat

~~~~~~

¾ c. corn flakes
½ small bagel, toasted
1 tsp. reduced-calorie margarine
1 c. skim milk
1 c. mixed melon cubes
Exchanges: 2 breads, 1 fruit, 1 milk

~~~~~~

½ c. cooked grits
1 tsp. reduced-calorie margarine
1 slice diet whole-wheat bread, toasted
1 tsp. all-fruit spread
1 small banana
1 c. skim milk
Exchanges: 2 breads, 1 fruit, 1 milk, ½ fat

~~~~~~

1 c. oatmeal
½ grapefruit
1 c. skim milk
Exchanges: 1 ½ breads, 1 fruit, 1 milk

~~~~~~

3 4-inch low-fat pancakes

1 tbsp. sugar-free syrup

1 c. strawberries, sliced

1 c. skim milk

Exchanges: 2 breads, 1 fruit, 1 milk, ½ fat

~~~~~~

1 c. fortified flake cereal

1 c. skim milk

1 small banana

Exchanges: 1 ½ breads, 1 fruit, 1 milk

~~~~~~

½ c. bran flakes

1 tbsp. raisins

1 c. milk

1 slice diet whole-wheat bread, toasted

1 tsp. all-fruit spread

Exchanges: 2 breads, ½ fruit, 1 milk

~~~~~~

Spanish Omelet

½ c. egg substitute

¼ c. tomatoes, diced

1 tsp. onions, diced

1 tsp. peppers, diced

   Nonstick cooking spray

Spray small frying pan with nonstick cooking spray. Combine ingredients and cook over medium heat until done.

Serve with 1 slice whole-wheat diet toast and ½ cup fresh pineapple.

Exchanges: 1 meat, 1 bread, ½ vegetable, 1 fruit

~~~~~~

1 2-oz. sesame bagel

1 tbsp. fat-free cream cheese

½ c. orange juice

6 oz. nonfat fruit-flavored yogurt

Exchanges: ½ meat, 2 breads, 1 fruit, 1 milk

~~~~~~

1 small reduced-fat blueberry muffin
1 c. skim milk
½ c. cinnamon applesauce
Exchanges: 2 breads, 1 fruit, 1 milk, ½ fat

~~~~~~

½ c. cooked grits
1 oz. 2% cheddar cheese, shredded
1 slice diet whole-wheat bread
1 tsp. all-fruit spread
½ c. orange juice
Exchanges: 1 meat, 2 breads, 1 fruit, ½ fat

~~~~~~

2 Eggo low-fat waffles
2 tsp. strawberry all-fruit spread
1 c. strawberries, sliced
1 c. skim milk
Exchanges: 2 breads, 1 fruit, 1 milk, ½ fat

~~~~~~

English Muffin Sandwich

1 English muffin
1 oz. Canadian bacon, sautéed
1 slice tomato
   Serve with 1 small orange.
Exchanges: 1 meat, 2 breads, 1 fruit

~~~~~~

☺ LUNCHES

1 c. all-vegetable soup (90-100 calories)
6 saltine crackers

~~~~~~

Tuna Sandwich

½ c. water-packed tuna
1 tbsp. reduced-fat mayonnaise
½ tsp. pickle relish
2 slices diet whole-wheat bread
   Lettuce and tomato
   Serve with 1 cup diced watermelon.
Exchanges: 2 meats, 2 breads, 1 vegetable, 1 fruit, ½ fat

~~~~~~

2 oz. turkey, sliced
1 · 2-oz. bagel, spread with
1 tsp. reduced-fat mayonnaise
Lettuce and tomato
1 c. carrot sticks
Serve with 1 apple.
Exchanges: 2 meats, 2 breads, 1 vegetable, 1 fruit

~ ~

1 c. tomato juice
1 c. celery sticks
6 slices Melba toast
½ c. 2% cottage cheese
⅓ c. peach slices
Exchanges: 2 meats, 1 ½ breads, 2 vegetables, 1 fruit

~ ~

Chick-fil-A Grilled Chicken Sandwich

Side of carrot and raisin salad
Serve with 15 red grapes.
Exchanges: 3 meats, 2 breads, 1 vegetable, 1 fruit, 1 fat

~ ~

Ham, Asparagus and Rice Rolls

2 oz. lean ham, sliced thin
4 large asparagus spears, cooked
½ c. cooked brown rice

Wrap ham around asparagus spears and rice.
Serve with 1 pear.
Exchanges: 2 meats, 1 ½ breads, 1 vegetable, 1 fruit

~ ~

Arby's Junior Roast Beef Sandwich

Dark green salad with veggies
1 tbsp. reduced-fat dressing
Serve with 1 small apple.
Exchanges: 2 meats, 2 breads, 1 vegetable, 1 fruit, 1 fat

~ ~

1   2-oz. sesame bagel, toasted
1   tsp. reduced-calorie margarine
½   c. 2% cottage cheese
½   c. fresh pineapple chunks
1   c. mixed carrot and celery sticks

Exchanges: 2 meats, 2 breads, 1 vegetable, 1 fruit, 1 fat

~~~~~~

Healthy Choice Linguini with Shrimp

Serve with ½ cup mixed-fruit salad.

Exchanges: 1 meat, 2 breads, 1 vegetable, 1 fruit

~~~~~~

2   tbsp. reduced-fat peanut butter
4   graham cracker squares
1   apple, sliced
1   c. broccoli florets

Exchanges: 1 meat, 1 bread, 1 vegetable, 1 fruit, 1 fat

~~~~~~

1   small low-fat granola bar
6   saltine crackers
2   oz. 2% cheddar cheese, sliced
4   canned apricot halves

Exchanges: 2 meats, 2 breads, 1 fruit, 1 fat

~~~~~~

Chef's Salad

1   oz. turkey, sliced in thin strips
1   oz. lean ham, sliced in thin strips
2   c. mixed salad greens
    Tomatoes, carrots and cucumbers
2   tbsp. reduced-fat dressing
Serve with 2 small bread sticks and 1 pear.

Exchanges: 2 meats, 2 breads, 1 vegetable, 1 fruit, ½ fat

~~~~~~

McDonald's Hamburger Happy Meal

Small diet drink
Green salad with fat-free dressing

Exchanges: 1½ meats, 3 breads, 1 vegetable, 1½ fats

~~~~~~

Stouffer's Lean Cuisine Fiesta Chicken

Dark green salad
Tomatoes, carrots and cucumbers
1   tbsp. reduced-fat dressing
Serve with 1 small orange.
Exchanges: 2 meats, 1 ½ breads, 1 ½ vegetables, 1 fruit, ½ fat

~ ~

Quesadillas

2   6-inch reduced-fat tortillas
2   oz. 2% cheddar cheese, shredded
½   c. salsa
¼   c. reduced-fat sour cream
Nonstick cooking spray

Coat medium skillet with nonstick cooking spray. Place half the cheese in each tortilla and fold in half. Cook over medium heat 2 minutes on each side.

Serve with 4 celery sticks with lite ranch dressing, salsa and sour cream.
Exchanges: 2 meats, 2 breads, 1 ½ vegetables, 1 fat

~ ~

🍎 DINNERS

Southwestern-Style Baked Fish with Black Bean Salsa

Salsa

1 16-oz. can black beans, drained
1 tbsp. red onion, diced
1 tsp. chili powder

1   c. chunky salsa
1   tbsp. fresh cilantro, chopped

Fish

4   4-oz. fish fillets
    (snapper, catfish, tilapia or grouper)
2   tsp. lime juice

Salt and black pepper
½   tsp. ground cumin
Nonstick cooking spray

For Salsa: Combine all ingredients in small bowl.
For Fish: Coat 9x9-inch baking pan with nonstick cooking spray. Season

fillets in pan and bake at 400° F for 12-15 minutes (10 minutes per inch of thickness). Garnish with salsa. Serves 4.

Serve each with ⅓ cup rice, one 6-inch ear of corn and 1 cup steamed broccoli with 1 teaspoon melted margarine.

Exchanges: 3 meats, 2½ breads, 1½ vegetables, 1 fat

~ ~

Spicy Eggplant Casserole

2	small eggplants, peeled and cut into 1-inch cubes
1½	tbsp. onion, chopped
1½	tbsp. celery, chopped
1½	tbsp. bell pepper, chopped
1	10-oz. can diced tomatoes with chilies
	Salt and cayenne pepper to taste
½	c. soft bread cubes
2	oz. 2% cheddar cheese, shredded
	Nonstick cooking spray

Salt eggplant and let sit 20 minutes to draw out bitterness. Rinse and drain. Combine eggplant and remaining ingredients, except for cheese, in bowl and pour into 9x9-inch baking dish coated with nonstick cooking spray. Top with cheese and bake at 400° F for 20-25 minutes. Serves 4.

Serve with a green salad with reduced-fat dressing and a bread stick.

Exchanges: ½ meat, 1 bread, 2 vegetables, ½ fat

~ ~

Vegetable Lasagna

6	no-bake lasagna noodles	2	eggs, slightly beaten
2	tbsp. canola oil	2	c. ricotta cheese
1	c. onion, chopped	4	tbsp. Parmesan cheese
1½	c. carrots, sliced thin	1	c. mushrooms, sliced
2	tsp. garlic, minced	1	tsp. leaf basil
1	15-oz. jar spaghetti sauce	½	tsp. leaf oregano
1	c. zucchini, quartered and sliced		Nonstick cooking spray
1	c. part-skim mozzarella cheese, shredded	1	10-oz. package frozen chopped spinach, thawed and drained

Heat oil in saucepan. Add onion, carrots and garlic. Sauté for 5-6 minutes or until tender. Add sauce and spices. Bring to a simmer. Blend eggs with ricotta cheese, Parmesan cheese and vegetables. Spread thin layer of sauce in bottom of a 9x13-inch baking pan coated with nonstick cooking spray. Cover with a layer of noodles. Spoon half the cheese-vegetable mixture over noodles. Cover with half of remaining sauce. Repeat. Cover with foil and bake at 350° F for 20 minutes. Remove foil and top with mozzarella cheese. Bake uncovered for 15 minutes. Let sit 10 minutes before slicing. Serves 6.

Serve each slice with a 3-inch slice of French bread with 1 teaspoon margarine, a tossed salad with reduced fat dressing, and a cup of fruit salad.
Exchanges: 3 meats, 2 breads, 2 vegetables, 1 fruit, 1 fat

~~~~~~

Chicken Cacciatore

1   2½-lb. chicken, quartered with skin removed
1   16-oz. can Italian-style tomatoes with peppers
1   onion, sliced
1   tsp. Italian herb seasoning
1   8-oz. can tomato sauce
2   c. frozen peas
     Nonstick cooking spray

Spray a large saucepan with nonstick cooking spray. Add chicken and remaining ingredients, except peas. Cover and simmer 25-35 minutes, stirring occasionally. Add peas and cook an additional 10 minutes. Serves 4.

Serve each with ½ cup boiled red potatoes and ½ cup steamed baby carrots.
Exchanges: 3 meats, 2 breads, 2 vegetables, ½ fat

~~~~~~

Stouffer's Beef Macaroni Casserole

Serve with a spinach salad with mushrooms and reduced-fat salad dressing and a peach.
Exchanges: 2 meats, 2 breads, 1 vegetable, 1 fruit, 1 fat

~~~~~~

Longhorn Chicken Kebob

Serve with a side salad with fat-free dressing and a side of rice and vegetables or stuffed potato with toppings on the side.
Exchanges: 3 meats, 2 breads, 1½ vegetable, 1 fat

~~~~~~

Grilled Hawaiian Chicken

4 4-oz. boneless chicken breasts
with skin
½ c. pineapple juice
¼ c. soy sauce
½ c. cooking sherry
1 tsp. brown sugar
8 fresh pineapple slices

Place chicken in a glass bowl. Combine remaining ingredients and pour over chicken breasts and marinate overnight or up to 48 hours. Remove breasts and grill over medium heat until done. Remove skin before serving. Grill fresh pineapple slices for garnish. Serves 4.

Serve each with ⅔ cup Uncle Ben's flavored rice pilaf and 1 cup sautéed snap peas.

Exchanges: 3 meats, 2 breads, 2 vegetables, 1 fruit

~ ~

Campbell's Chunky Manhattan-Style Clam Chowder

Dark green salad

Cucumbers, carrots and tomatoes

Fat-free dressing

Exchanges: 3 breads, 1 vegetable, 2 fats

~ ~

Chicken Ratatouille

4 4-oz. boneless, skinless
chicken breasts, cubed
1 large tomato, cubed
½ tsp. leaf thyme
1 tsp. leaf basil
½ tsp. granulated garlic
green bell pepper, sliced
½ lb. mushrooms, sliced
1 tbsp. olive oil
1 small eggplant, cubed
2 small zucchini, sliced
1 onion, sliced
1 tsp. black pepper

In a large saucepan, sauté chicken in olive oil (about 2 minutes per side). Add eggplant, zucchini, onion, mushrooms and bell pepper. Simmer 10 minutes. Add tomato and remaining ingredients. Simmer 3-5 minutes. Serves 4.

Serve each with ⅔ cup cooked rice and a Caesar salad with low-fat dressing.

Exchanges: 3 meats, 2 breads, 2 vegetables, 1 fat

~ ~

Grilled or Broiled Halibut

4 4-oz. halibut filets
2 tbsp. lite Italian dressing
2 tsp. Worcestershire sauce

½ tsp. paprika
¼ tsp. black pepper

In a 9x9-inch dish, combine all ingredients. Let marinate for 30 minutes in refrigerator. Grill or broil fish about 10 minutes per inch of thickness (about 5 minutes per side).

Serve each with ½ cup mashed potatoes, 1 cup assorted grilled vegetables and a dinner roll.

Exchanges: 3 meats, 2 breads, 1 vegetable, ½ fat

~~~~~~

Beef Kebobs

1 lb. lean sirloin, cut into 1-inch cubes
1 small red onion, quartered
1 green bell pepper, cut into 1-inch pieces
8 mushroom caps
1 zucchini, cut into 12 rounds

2 tsp. olive oil
2 tsp. Worcestershire sauce
½ tsp. leaf oregano
¼ tsp. black pepper
12 cherry tomatoes

Alternate meat and vegetables, except cherry tomatoes, on a wooden or metal skewer. Place in a glass dish. In a small bowl combine oil, Worcestershire sauce, oregano and pepper. Pour over kebabs and let marinate covered in refrigerator overnight. Grill to desired doneness and garnish with cherry tomatoes.

Serve each with ½ cup grilled red potatoes, a slice of toasted French bread and ½ cup boiled baby carrots sprayed with butter-flavored cooking spray.

Exchanges: 3 meats, 2 breads, 2 vegetables, ½ fat

~~~~~~

Turkey Steak

4 3-oz. turkey mignons
1 tsp. canola oil
2 tsp. lemon-pepper seasoning

½ c. reduced-fat ranch dressing
1 tbsp. brown mustard
¼ tsp. dried dill

Heat oil in large pan. Add mignons and sauté over medium heat 8-10 minutes, turning occasionally. Add lemon-pepper seasoning and sauté 1 minute more on each side. Combine remaining ingredients to use as a sauce.

Serve each with 1 cup steamed cauliflower topped with small amount of sauce and one serving of prepared herbed stuffing mix.
Exchanges: 2½ meats, 2 breads, 1 vegetable, ½ fat

~~~~~~

Shrimp and Vegetable Risotto

¾ lb. precooked salad shrimp
2 tbsp. olive oil, divided
6 plum tomatoes, quartered and seeded
1 medium zucchini, cubed
1 medium summer squash, cubed
1 c. mushrooms, sliced
1 c. onions, chopped

1 clove garlic, minced
1 tsp. leaf oregano
3 c. chicken broth
¾ c. Arborio rice
¼ c. Parmesan cheese, grated
Salt and pepper
½ c. frozen peas, thawed

Heat oil in large pan. Add vegetables and sauté over medium heat until crisp tender. Add shrimp and keep warm. In a separate saucepan, add oregano, broth and rice. Bring to a boil. Simmer until thickened, stirring occasionally. Stir in Parmesan cheese and season with salt and pepper. In a large bowl, combine shrimp mixture with rice mixture. Toss and garnish with peas. Serves 4.

Serve with toasted pita chips.
Exchanges: 3 meats, 2 breads, 1½ vegetables, ½ fat

~~~~~~

Pasta Primavera with Meat Sauce

6 oz. uncooked penne pasta
¾ lb. extra lean ground beef
¼ c. onion, diced
¼ c. bell pepper, diced
1 10-oz. package frozen stir-fry vegetables, thawed

1 tsp. granulated garlic
1 tsp. salt
3 c. prepared spaghetti sauce
1 c. mushrooms, sliced
1 tbsp. shredded Parmesan cheese
Nonstick cooking spray

Cook pasta according to package directions, omitting fat and salt. Drain and set aside. In a large saucepan sprayed with nonstick cooking spray, sauté onion and bell pepper. Add mushrooms, garlic, salt and ground beef. Cook until done, about 12 minutes. Drain off excess fat. Add sauce and vegetables and simmer for an additional 5 minutes. Serve on top of pasta and garnish with Parmesan. Serves 4.

Serve with a green salad and bread sticks.
Exchanges: 3 meats, 2 breads, 2 vegetables, ½ fat

CONVERSION CHART
EQUIVALENT IMPERIAL AND METRIC MEASUREMENTS

Liquid Measures

Fluid Ounces	U.S.	Imperial	Milliliters
	1 teaspoon	1 teaspoon	5
$\frac{1}{4}$	2 teaspoons	1 dessert spoon	7
$\frac{1}{2}$	1 tablespoon	1 tablespoon	15
1	2 tablespoons	2 tablespoons	28
2	$\frac{1}{4}$ cup	4 tablespoons	56
4	$\frac{1}{2}$ cup or $\frac{1}{4}$ pint		110
5		$\frac{1}{4}$ pint or 1 gill	140
6	$\frac{3}{4}$ cup		170
8	1 cup or $\frac{1}{2}$ pint		225
9			250 or $\frac{1}{4}$ liter
10	$1\frac{1}{4}$ cups	$\frac{1}{2}$ pint	280
12	$1\frac{1}{2}$ cups or $\frac{3}{4}$ pint		340
15		3/4 pint	420
16	2 cups or 1 pint		450
18	$2\frac{1}{4}$ cups		500 or $\frac{1}{2}$ liter
20	$2\frac{1}{2}$ cups	1 pint	560
24	3 cups or $1\frac{1}{2}$ pints		675
25		$1\frac{1}{4}$	700
30	$3\frac{3}{4}$ cups	$1\frac{1}{2}$ pints	840
32	4 cups		900
36	$4\frac{1}{2}$ cups		1000 or 1 liter
40	5 cups	2 pints or 1 quart	1120
48	6 cups or 3 pints		1350
50		$2\frac{1}{2}$ pints	1400

Solid Measures

U.S. and Imperial Measures		Metric Measures	
Ounces	Pounds	Grams	Kilos
1		28	
2		56	
3½		100	
4	¼	112	
5		140	
6		168	
8	½	225	
9		250	¼
12	¾	340	
16	1	450	
18		500	½
20	1¼	560	
24	1½	675	
27		750	¾
32	2	900	
36	2¼	1000	1
40	2½	1100	
48	3	1350	
54		1500	1½
64	4	1800	
72	4½	2000	2
80	5	2250	2¼
100	6	2800	2¾

Oven Temperature Equivalents

Fahrenheit	Celcius	Gas Mark	Description
225	110	$\frac{1}{4}$	Cool
250	130	$\frac{1}{2}$	
275	140	1	Very Slow
300	150	2	
325	170	3	Slow
350	180	4	Moderate
375	190	5	
400	200	6	Moderately Hot
425	220	7	Fairly Hot
450	230	8	Hot
475	240	9	Very Hot
500	250	10	Extremely Hot

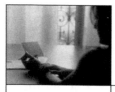

LEADER'S DISCUSSION GUIDE

Week One: Seeking God's Best

1. Say the memory verse, John 6:35, in unison. Discuss: Since Jesus said He would meet our needs if we come to Him, why are so many Christians unsatisfied in life?

2. Remind members that sharing is voluntary and confidentiality is important. Ask volunteers to share the changes God has already made in their lives. Remind members that the same God who saved them will continue to meet their needs. Read Philippians 4:19. Discuss the difference between needs and wants.

3. Point out that the opposite of being nourished is experiencing a drought where food and water are in short supply. Have members form groups of three to discuss the contrast between spiritual drought and spiritual nourishment (Day 2). Bring the whole group back together to report a summary of their discussions. After the groups report, stress the importance of staying with the basic commitments of prayer and Bible study as the way to sustain their spiritual lives.

4. Invite group members to share an unpleasant circumstance during which they were able to be content and the character trait that God strengthened during that time. Have groups conclude by thanking God for the difficulties in their lives that make them grow.

5. Discuss the importance of keeping the nine commitments of First Place. Affirm the importance of the commitment of being an encouragement and source of joy to one another and a witness of God's power in their lives.

6. Review members' definitions of a committed heart from 1 Kings 8:61. Suggested answers might include a life that is purposeful, contented, disciplined and obedient to God's plan.

7. Discuss using the memory verse in prayer. Close with a prayer asking God to satisfy members' needs. Incorporate the memory verse into your prayer.

Week Two: Committed to Returning

1. Invite volunteers to say the memory verse. Ask if anyone can repeat last week's verse. Invite someone to name the five steps (from the titles of each day's study) necessary to returning to God's blessings.

2. **Before the meeting,** enlist a group member to share a testimony that demonstrates the benefits of embracing change, even when it takes us out of our comfort zones. Discuss: What fears hinder people from making changes God wants them to make (e.g., fear of failure, fear of the unknown, fear of rejection, fear of financial loss, etc.)? Which of these fears might apply to our goals in First Place? After a couple of minutes of discussion, call on the group member you enlisted to give a testimony.

3. Remind members of the stress we put on ourselves when we don't take time to seek God's way of doing something. Contrast God's timing with ours. Let members share times when God delayed an answer to prayer, but when the answer came, they could see that God's timing was best.

4. Brainstorm characteristics of people in general who are difficult to love. Warn members *not* to mention specific names of difficult people in their lives—just speak in general terms. Discuss the need to see people as God sees them. Have members use their study book to write a private list of people that they need to ask God to help them love. Have a silent time of prayer for these difficult people. End the discussion with a testimony about a difficult person whom God eventually used to bless your life.

5. Display a picture of a maze or discuss what a maze is. Compare finding God's will to the difficulty of finding the way out of a maze. Explain: A maze is easier to negotiate when we know the designer has provided a way out. We can also use the knowledge we gained from successfully completing other mazes. Make spiritual parallels to these points.

6. Refer to the description of worship from Day 4 found in John 4:21-24 (p. 27). Invite members to share about times they have experienced true worship. Share ideas and helps for private worship and how to encourage family and corporate worship in church.

7. Invite a volunteer to share his or her salvation experience. Tell the group that you are available if anyone would like to learn more about accepting Christ's salvation. Close with short sentence prayers of thanksgiving for God's salvation.

Week Three: Welcome Home

1. Say in unison 1 Thessalonians 5:18. Invite members to say one-sentence praises for a difficult circumstance God is using as a blessing in their lives.

2. Discuss the question from Day 1 (p. 35) about a personal experience of returning to a group or place after a long absence. Invite members to share memories of the reactions to their homecoming. Ask them to silently reflect on a time when they felt they returned to the Lord after a time of distance from Him. Emphasize the fact that God always greets us with joy and celebration. We need never fear returning to Him.

3. Read Hebrews 10:24-25. Discuss ways Christians can encourage each other spiritually and in health and fitness goals. Affirm someone who has been an encourager to you in First Place. Allow volunteers to affirm those in the group who have been encouragers to them. Suggest ways members can fulfill the encouragement commitment of First Place (e.g., cards, phone calls, e-mails, personal encounters, etc.).

4. Review Naomi's request to be called Mara, or "bitter" (p. 36). Display or show a picture of a basket of fresh apples. Ask members what will happen if you put a rotten apple in the basket. Compare a bitter person's influence on those around him or her with the ability of a rotten apple to spoil other apples. Invite responses to the meaning of Hebrews 12:14-15 (p. 37).

5. Form small groups. Have groups share and discuss three things: (1) a hurtful personal experience from which God received glory, (2) possible reasons God may have allowed these difficulties, and (3) ways to weather difficult times without becoming bitter.

6. Guide a time for members to pray silently, naming hurts and difficulties they need to release to God. Then lead a prayer of surrender, yielding those hurts to the Lord.

7. Challenge members to be encouragers this week by affirming each other verbally. Remind them to pray for specific hurts and needs were mentioned.

Week Four: Beginning a Love Relationship

1. Repeat the memory verse, Titus 2:13-14. Invite a volunteer to repeat the verses from weeks one, two or three. Discuss: What is the blessed

hope mentioned in verse 13? What has God redeemed you from? What does "purified" mean? Lead members to discuss some good deeds that are outgrowths of a pure lifestyle.

2. Review Ruth's divine appointment from Day 1. Ask volunteers to share divine appointments from their lives.

3. Form small groups and invite individuals to share times when, like Ruth, they felt like an outsider (Day 2). Discuss the acceptance Christ gives us when we come to Him. Contrast the unconditional love of God with the world's idea of love and acceptance.

4. Distribute paper to each small group. Instruct members to compile a master list from their descriptions of life to the full from John 10:10 (p. 51). Have groups post these on the walls and read them aloud to the other groups when you call for reports. Challenge members to experience the abundant life they described.

5. **Before the meeting**, obtain a genealogical chart found in a family Bible or other source. Reconvene the whole group. Display the genealogical chart. Invite volunteers to tell something about an ancestor that the group would find interesting or amusing. Point out that Jesus is in our family tree. We are His heirs! Brainstorm what we receive from our inheritance in Him.

6. From the list they compiled on Day 5 (p. 53), have members pray silently for persons who need to be included in God's family. Lead a spoken prayer for members to move beyond their salvation experience to join God in His work in the world.

7. Close by reading together Matthew 28:19-20.

Week Five: Qualities Pleasing to God

1. Review the memory verse. Ask members to give examples of the way God views things that differ from the ways we look at the same things.

2. Have members name ways kindness can open doors for sharing the love of Christ. Have them share times when God used someone's kind deed to encourage them. Discuss: Why are kindness and forgiveness linked in Ephesians 4:32?

3. Form small groups and have them discuss characteristics of spiritually mature people that they listed on Day 2. Point out that discerning God's Spirit and speaking His truth are essential elements of Christian

spirituality. Being a good person is not enough. Remind them that spiritual discernment can only be given by God.

4. Reconvene the whole group. Invite volunteers to tell how a first impression proved wrong concerning a person that they had met. Discuss: Is it fair to judge someone by his or her appearance? Refer to the memory verse as an example of the way God judges us. Discuss: What kind of qualities should we look for in a spiritually mature person? Mention the traits discussed in 1 Peter 3:3-4, such as a gentle and quiet spirit.

5. Discuss: How is the idea of having a servant's heart different from the prevailing selfishness in the world today? Why is it difficult to have a servant's heart? Have members brainstorm ways they can serve others through their participation in the First Place program.

6. Discuss: What are synonyms for the word "diligent"? Point out the importance of following through as in sports—such as swinging a golf club, hitting a baseball, making a jump shot or throwing a bowling ball—reminding them about the importance of follow-through in our spiritual lives. Remind them that spiritual diligence means they follow through with their commitments to the Lord.

7. Pray for God to help each of them follow through on his or her commitment to the Lord and to the First Place program.

Week Six: Protecting Your Relationship

1. Repeat this week's memory verse in unison. Discuss ways members have resisted Satan in their First Place commitments during the week. Invite someone to explain how submitting to God is a key to resisting Satan.

2. Form five small groups. Assign each group one of the five days of study to review. Give members the following assignment written on a white board, newsprint or poster board: As you review your portion of the study, (1) name reasons we need protection in this area of our lives; (2) name ways we can seek protection; (3) share Scripture verses to encourage or instruct us in this area of our lives.

   After five to seven minutes, reconvene the whole group. Invite small groups to report their key ideas. Be prepared to summarize each group's key points. Encourage members to associate with positive people who are spiritual encouragers and to permeate their minds with uplifting Christian music, words and visual images. Discuss the power of advertising and its influence.

3. In regard to protecting our time (Day 3), discuss: How does busyness interfere with our priorities for exercise, nutritious eating and Bible study?

4. **Before the meeting,** gather several sticks or small branches. Demonstrate the difference between breaking one thin stick and breaking several sticks tied together. Emphasize the importance of the strength we gain when we have Christian friends who surround us with prayer and accountability.

5. Read the case study of Hank from Day 5 (p. 77). Discuss: What usually happens when we let down our guard? Remind members of the armor of God necessary for our protection (see Ephesians 6:10-18).

6. Invite members to pray silently concerning one area of temptation for which they need God's protection. Then lead a closing prayer for God's protection for your group.

Week Seven: In God's Hands

1. Invite several members to repeat the memory verse for the week. Discuss: What does this truth say to those who worry about the future? How does believing in God's provision affect your joy?

2. Invite volunteers to share ways God protects us. Remind members of the many times we take His protection for granted. Compare our protective care from God to a newborn who is not aware of all the ways his or her parents are providing for and protecting him or her. In the same way, we are not aware of all the provisions and protection our heavenly Father constantly gives us. However, we should note and express thanks for those of which we are aware.

    Explain: Gratefulness cannot exist if we constantly feel we deserve more. Encourage members to express thankfulness for little things God has provided. Remind them that a person who is truly grateful for God's provision is a joyous, positive and delightful companion. Discuss how a grateful person is a better testimony for the Lord than a worrying, pessimistic, complaining one.

3. Form small groups and assign the following questions based on Day 3. Display these questions on a white board, newsprint or poster board or write them on sheets of paper in advance for each group.

- What things make people feel unacceptable to others and to God?

- How can you help those who feel inadequate feel accepted?

- How important is a person's self-worth to success in maintaining a healthy lifestyle?

- What Bible verses remind us of our importance and worth to God?

4. Reconvene the whole group and ask for each group's report.

5. Brainstorm ways you can serve God through your work inside or outside the home. Discuss: What difference should it make when we work as though God is our boss?

6. Have small groups of two or three share a word of affirmation to each other and then pray for ways they might serve the Lord by serving others this week.

Week Eight: Preparing for God's Best

1. Review the memory verse for the week. Ask members to share synonyms for the word "consecrate."

2. **Before the meeting,** prepare five large footprints—the size of a man's shoe—made out of paper on which you have written the five steps studied this week: (1) Don't settle for less. (2) Do your spiritual homework. (3) Exercise faith. (4) Act in obedience. (5) Claim the blessing. Display the footprints around the room. Remind members that all the five steps are important in experiencing God's blessings. Have them share reasons people avoid cleansing their lives with God (i.e., removing barriers to their relationship). Discuss: What influences in our world keep us from being consecrated?

3. Read Acts 1:8. Discuss the power of God demonstrated by these early followers of Christ. Explain that we have the same power to overcome sin in our lives today. However, there is a direct relationship between the power of God in us and our level of consecration to Him.

4. Compare a Christian who doesn't continue in commitment to the Lord to a partially followed recipe, an incomplete map, an unfinished garment or an unfinished term paper. Explain: These items are not very useful if not completed. Discuss: What is the key to continuing? (Consistent abiding in His presence and obedience to His Word.)

5. **Before the meeting,** prepare a wrapped gift. Discuss: How would we appreciate this gift? Explain: We can't claim promises we don't know. God wants us to know His Word. Invite members to share promises in Scripture that reveal His blessings for us. Write responses on the board. Have the group review the list to determine how many depend on our obedience.

6. Remind members that Jesus called obedience the highest expression of love (see John 14:15). Ask the group to silently reflect on any unconfessed sin for which they need to ask forgiveness, and express a willingness to follow all the steps necessary for God's power and blessings on their lives.

Week Nine: Standing on the Promises

1. Review the memory verse for the week. Give a personal testimony, **or before the meeting,** ask a member to prepare to give an example of the truth that "your labor in the Lord is not in vain." Invite a volunteer to recite all nine verses memorized thus far in the study.

2. Brainstorm biblical principles that model Christian business practices (e.g., the Ten Commandments and the Golden Rule). Discuss the straightforward way that Boaz conducted business at the city gate.

3. Discuss how Jesus is our kinsman-redeemer because He bought us out of slavery to sin and made us heirs in His family. Invite volunteers to list some of the concerns that brought them to First Place (p. 107). Encourage members to give their concerns to Jesus, our kinsman-redeemer and provider.

4. Read and discuss Matthew 19:29. Explain that the meaning has more to do with priorities than abandonment of family. Invite them to share instances when they have seen family ties keep people from serving the Lord.

5. Display an object, such as a ring, that has greatly increased in worth over the years. Perhaps the value is sentimental as well as material. Compare this increase in value to the riches we receive in Christ when we pay the price of yielding to Him as Lord. Whatever we give Him, He multiplies and gives back.

6. Encourage members to be prayer warriors for one another. Distribute paper or inexpensive stationery and envelopes. Give members an opportunity to write a note of encouragement and then pray silently

for someone on their prayer list. Encourage them to mail the note during the coming week.

7. Sing songs of praise and thanksgiving. Have individuals share one sentence praises. Close with prayer.

Week Ten: The Blessings from God

1. Discuss the promises given in Psalm 23:5-6. Discuss: When God rewards your efforts in First Place with a physically fit body, how could you give Him glory? Suggest other blessings God may have given as a result of this study and ways we can give God glory for them.

2. Invite volunteers to name the blessings of each of the major characters from the book of Ruth. Discuss: How difficult is it to have faith in the midst of trials? What spiritual truths from the book of Ruth could help you during these trials? Can you thank God in the midst of these trials for the character He is building in your life?

3. Form small groups. Review Galatians 6:9 from Day 2. Invite members to share (1) a time when they quit on a project and later realized they should have stayed with it—i.e., piano lessons, a witnessing program or a job opportunity; and (2) times they were discouraged, yet God enabled them to continue with their goals.

   After five to seven minutes of small group discussion, reconvene the whole group and explain that at times rest can help us recharge and get a new perspective on our goals. Sometimes we neglect exercise or good eating habits because of fatigue. Rest is the solution to the problem. After a period of rest, exercise may seem more desirable and food less desirable.

4. Invite members to reflect silently on the characteristics of Naomi, Ruth and Boaz that they might need to develop in their own lives. Invite volunteers to share their list of characteristics.

5. Lead members to express what this study has meant to them in terms of identifying and seeking God's best. Invite volunteers to share methods they have used to help them memorize the Bible verses each week. Ask members to share a memory verse that had special meaning for them during this session.

6. Invite volunteers to pray, asking God for continued victories in their lives; or ask members to choose a memory verse and repeat it in the form of a prayer. Close with hugs or other appropriate symbols of parting.

PERSONAL WEIGHT RECORD

Week	Weight	+ or -	Goal This Session	Pounds to Goal
1				
2				
3				
4				
5				
6				
7				
8				
9				
10				
11				
12				
13				
Final				

Beginning Measurements

Waist_____ Hips_____ Thighs_____ Chest_____

Ending Measurements

Waist_____ Hips_____ Thighs_____ Chest_____

COMMITMENT RECORDS

How to Fill Out a Commitment Record

The Commitment Record (CR) is an aid for you in keeping track of your accomplishments. Begin a new CR on the morning of the day your class meets. This ensures that your CR is complete before your next meeting. Turn in the CR weekly to your leader.

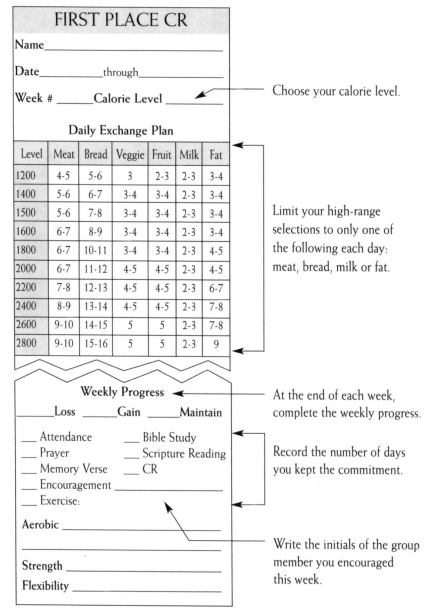

FIRST PLACE CR

Name_____

Date_____through_____

Week # _____Calorie Level _____ — Choose your calorie level.

Daily Exchange Plan

Level	Meat	Bread	Veggie	Fruit	Milk	Fat
1200	4-5	5-6	3	2-3	2-3	3-4
1400	5-6	6-7	3-4	3-4	2-3	3-4
1500	5-6	7-8	3-4	3-4	2-3	3-4
1600	6-7	8-9	3-4	3-4	2-3	3-4
1800	6-7	10-11	3-4	3-4	2-3	4-5
2000	6-7	11-12	4-5	4-5	2-3	4-5
2200	7-8	12-13	4-5	4-5	2-3	6-7
2400	8-9	13-14	4-5	4-5	2-3	7-8
2600	9-10	14-15	5	5	2-3	7-8
2800	9-10	15-16	5	5	2-3	9

Limit your high-range selections to only one of the following each day: meat, bread, milk or fat.

Weekly Progress — At the end of each week, complete the weekly progress.

_____Loss _____Gain _____Maintain

___ Attendance   ___ Bible Study
___ Prayer   ___ Scripture Reading
___ Memory Verse   ___ CR
___ Encouragement _____
___ Exercise:

Aerobic _____

_____

Strength _____

Flexibility _____

Record the number of days you kept the commitment.

Write the initials of the group member you encouraged this week.

DAY 7:   Date _____

Morning _____
_____
_____

Midday _____
_____
_____

Evening _____
_____
_____

Snacks _____
_____
_____

___ **Meat** _____   ☐ Prayer
___ **Bread** _____   ☐ Bible Study
___ **Vegetable** ____   ☐ Scripture Reading
___ **Fruit** _____   ☐ Memory Verse
___ **Milk** _____   ☐ Encouragement
___ **Fat** _____   ☐ Water_____

Exercise:
Aerobic _____
_____
Strength _____
Flexibility _____

List the foods you have eaten. On this condensed CR it is not necessary to exchange each food choice. It will be the responsibility of each member that the tally marks you list below are accurate regarding each food choice. If you are unsure of an exchange, check the Live-It section of your copy of the *Member's Guide*.

List the daily food exchange choices to the left of the food groups.

Use tally marks for the actual food and water consumed.

Check off commitments completed. Use tally marks to record each 8-oz. serving of water.

List type and duration of exercise.

Name _____

Date _____ through _____

Week # _____ **Calorie Level** _____

Daily Exchange Plan

Level	Meat	Bread	Veggie	Fruit	Milk	Fat
1200	4-5	5-6	3	2-3	2-3	3-4
1400	5-6	6-7	3-4	3-4	2-3	3-4
1500	5-6	7-8	3-4	3-4	2-3	3-4
1600	6-7	8-9	3-4	3-4	2-3	3-4
1800	6-7	10-11	3-4	3-4	2-3	4-5
2000	6-7	11-12	4-5	4-5	2-3	4-5
2200	7-8	12-13	4-5	4-5	2-3	6-7
2400	8-9	13-14	4-5	4-5	2-3	7-8
2600	9-10	14-15	5	5	2-3	7-8
2800	9-10	15-16	5	5	2-3	9

You may always choose the high range of vegetables and fruits. Limit your high range selections to only one of the following: meat, bread, milk or fat.

Weekly Progress

_____ Loss _____ Gain _____ Maintain

_____ Attendance _____ Bible Study
_____ Prayer _____ Scripture Reading
_____ Memory Verse _____ CR
_____ Encouragement: _____
_____ Exercise _____
Aerobic _____

Strength _____
Flexibility _____

DAY 5: Date _____

Morning _____

Midday _____

Evening _____

Snacks _____

_____ Meat   ☐ Prayer
_____ Bread   ☐ Bible Study
_____ Vegetable ☐ Scripture Reading
_____ Fruit   ☐ Memory Verse
_____ Milk   ☐ Encouragement
_____ Fat   ☐ Water

Exercise
Aerobic _____

Strength _____
Flexibility _____

DAY 6: Date _____

Morning _____

Midday _____

Evening _____

Snacks _____

_____ Meat   ☐ Prayer
_____ Bread   ☐ Bible Study
_____ Vegetable ☐ Scripture Reading
_____ Fruit   ☐ Memory Verse
_____ Milk   ☐ Encouragement
_____ Fat   ☐ Water

Exercise
Aerobic _____

Strength _____
Flexibility _____

DAY 7: Date _____

Morning _____

Midday _____

Evening _____

Snacks _____

_____ Meat   ☐ Prayer
_____ Bread   ☐ Bible Study
_____ Vegetable ☐ Scripture Reading
_____ Fruit   ☐ Memory Verse
_____ Milk   ☐ Encouragement
_____ Fat   ☐ Water

Exercise
Aerobic _____

Strength _____
Flexibility _____

DAY 1: Date _____

Morning _____

Midday _____

Evening _____

Snacks _____

- ___ Meat _____   ☐ Prayer
- ___ Bread _____   ☐ Bible Study
- ___ Vegetable _____   ☐ Scripture Reading
- ___ Fruit _____   ☐ Memory Verse
- ___ Milk _____   ☐ Encouragement
- ___ Fat _____   ___ Water _____

Exercise

Aerobic _____

Strength _____

Flexibility _____

DAY 2: Date _____

Morning _____

Midday _____

Evening _____

Snacks _____

- ___ Meat _____   ☐ Prayer
- ___ Bread _____   ☐ Bible Study
- ___ Vegetable _____   ☐ Scripture Reading
- ___ Fruit _____   ☐ Memory Verse
- ___ Milk _____   ☐ Encouragement
- ___ Fat _____   ___ Water _____

Exercise

Aerobic _____

Strength _____

Flexibility _____

DAY 3: Date _____

Morning _____

Midday _____

Evening _____

Snacks _____

- ___ Meat _____   ☐ Prayer
- ___ Bread _____   ☐ Bible Study
- ___ Vegetable _____   ☐ Scripture Reading
- ___ Fruit _____   ☐ Memory Verse
- ___ Milk _____   ☐ Encouragement
- ___ Fat _____   ___ Water _____

Exercise

Aerobic _____

Strength _____

Flexibility _____

DAY 4: Date _____

Morning _____

Midday _____

Evening _____

Snacks _____

- ___ Meat _____   ☐ Prayer
- ___ Bread _____   ☐ Bible Study
- ___ Vegetable _____   ☐ Scripture Reading
- ___ Fruit _____   ☐ Memory Verse
- ___ Milk _____   ☐ Encouragement
- ___ Fat _____   ___ Water _____

Exercise

Aerobic _____

Strength _____

Flexibility _____

Name _____

Date _____ through _____

Week # _____ Calorie Level _____

Daily Exchange Plan

Level	Meat	Bread	Veggie	Fruit	Milk	Fat
1200	4-5	5-6	3	2-3	2-3	3-4
1400	5-6	6-7	3-4	3-4	2-3	3-4
1500	5-6	7-8	3-4	3-4	2-3	3-4
1600	6-7	8-9	3-4	3-4	2-3	3-4
1800	6-7	10-11	3-4	3-4	2-3	4-5
2000	6-7	11-12	4-5	4-5	2-3	4-5
2200	7-8	12-13	4-5	4-5	2-3	6-7
2400	8-9	13-14	4-5	4-5	2-3	7-8
2600	9-10	14-15	5	5	2-3	7-8
2800	9-10	15-16	5	5	2-3	9

You may always choose the high range of vegetables and fruits. Limit your high range selections to only one of the following: meat, bread, milk or fat.

_____ Loss _____ Gain _____ Maintain

_____ Attendance _____ Bible Study
_____ Prayer _____ Scripture Reading
_____ Memory Verse _____ CR
_____ Encouragement
_____ Exercise
Aerobic _____
Strength _____
Flexibility _____

DAY 5: Date _____

Morning _____

Midday _____

Evening _____

Snacks _____

_____ Meat   ☐ Prayer
_____ Bread   ☐ Bible Study
_____ Vegetable ☐ Scripture Reading
_____ Fruit   ☐ Memory Verse
_____ Milk   ☐ Encouragement
_____ Fat   _____ Water

Exercise
Aerobic _____

Strength _____
Flexibility _____

DAY 6: Date _____

Morning _____

Midday _____

Evening _____

Snacks _____

_____ Meat   ☐ Prayer
_____ Bread   ☐ Bible Study
_____ Vegetable ☐ Scripture Reading
_____ Fruit   ☐ Memory Verse
_____ Milk   ☐ Encouragement
_____ Fat   _____ Water

Exercise
Aerobic _____

Strength _____
Flexibility _____

DAY 7: Date _____

Morning _____

Midday _____

Evening _____

Snacks _____

_____ Meat   ☐ Prayer
_____ Bread   ☐ Bible Study
_____ Vegetable ☐ Scripture Reading
_____ Fruit   ☐ Memory Verse
_____ Milk   ☐ Encouragement
_____ Fat   _____ Water

Exercise
Aerobic _____

Strength _____
Flexibility _____

DAY 1: Date_____

Morning _____

Midday _____

Evening _____

Snacks _____

___ Meat	☐ Prayer
___ Bread	☐ Bible Study
___ Vegetable	☐ Scripture Reading
___ Fruit	☐ Memory Verse
___ Milk	☐ Encouragement
___ Fat	___ Water

Exercise
Aerobic _____

Strength _____
Flexibility _____

DAY 2: Date_____

Morning _____

Midday _____

Evening _____

Snacks _____

___ Meat	☐ Prayer
___ Bread	☐ Bible Study
___ Vegetable	☐ Scripture Reading
___ Fruit	☐ Memory Verse
___ Milk	☐ Encouragement
___ Fat	___ Water

Exercise
Aerobic _____

Strength _____
Flexibility _____

DAY 3: Date_____

Morning _____

Midday _____

Evening _____

Snacks _____

___ Meat	☐ Prayer
___ Bread	☐ Bible Study
___ Vegetable	☐ Scripture Reading
___ Fruit	☐ Memory Verse
___ Milk	☐ Encouragement
___ Fat	___ Water

Exercise
Aerobic _____

Strength _____
Flexibility _____

DAY 4: Date_____

Morning _____

Midday _____

Evening _____

Snacks _____

___ Meat	☐ Prayer
___ Bread	☐ Bible Study
___ Vegetable	☐ Scripture Reading
___ Fruit	☐ Memory Verse
___ Milk	☐ Encouragement
___ Fat	___ Water

Exercise
Aerobic _____

Strength _____
Flexibility _____

Name _____

Date _____ through _____

Week # _____ Calorie Level _____

Daily Exchange Plan

Level	Meat	Bread	Veggie	Fruit	Milk	Fat
1200	4-5	5-6	3	2-3	2-3	3-4
1400	5-6	6-7	3-4	3-4	2-3	3-4
1500	5-6	7-8	3-4	3-4	2-3	3-4
1600	6-7	8-9	3-4	3-4	2-3	3-4
1800	6-7	10-11	3-4	3-4	2-3	4-5
2000	6-7	11-12	4-5	4-5	2-3	4-5
2200	7-8	12-13	4-5	4-5	2-3	6-7
2400	8-9	13-14	4-5	4-5	2-3	7-8
2600	9-10	14-15	5	5	2-3	7-8
2800	9-10	15-16	5	5	2-3	9

You may always choose the high range of vegetables and fruits. Limit your high range selections to only one of the following: meat, bread, milk or fat.

_____ Loss _____ Gain _____ Maintain

_____ Attendance _____ Bible Study
_____ Prayer _____ Scripture Reading
_____ Memory Verse _____ CR
_____ Encouragement
_____ Exercise
Aerobic _____

Strength _____
Flexibility _____

DAY 5: Date _____

Morning _____
_____

Midday _____
_____

Evening _____
_____

Snacks _____
_____

_____ Meat _____
_____ Bread _____
_____ Vegetable _____
_____ Fruit _____
_____ Milk _____
_____ Fat _____
Exercise
Aerobic _____

Strength _____
Flexibility _____

☐ Prayer
☐ Bible Study
☐ Scripture Reading
☐ Memory Verse
☐ Encouragement
_____ Water

DAY 6: Date _____

Morning _____
_____

Midday _____
_____

Evening _____
_____

Snacks _____
_____

_____ Meat _____
_____ Bread _____
_____ Vegetable _____
_____ Fruit _____
_____ Milk _____
_____ Fat _____
Exercise
Aerobic _____

Strength _____
Flexibility _____

☐ Prayer
☐ Bible Study
☐ Scripture Reading
☐ Memory Verse
☐ Encouragement
_____ Water

DAY 7: Date _____

Morning _____
_____

Midday _____
_____

Evening _____
_____

Snacks _____
_____

_____ Meat _____
_____ Bread _____
_____ Vegetable _____
_____ Fruit _____
_____ Milk _____
_____ Fat _____
Exercise
Aerobic _____

Strength _____
Flexibility _____

☐ Prayer
☐ Bible Study
☐ Scripture Reading
☐ Memory Verse
☐ Encouragement
_____ Water

DAY 1: Date _____

Morning _____

Midday _____

Evening _____

Snacks _____

___ Meat	___ Bread	___ Vegetable	___ Fruit	___ Milk	___ Fat
☐ Prayer	☐ Bible Study	☐ Scripture Reading	☐ Memory Verse	☐ Encouragement	___ Water

Exercise
Aerobic _____
Strength _____
Flexibility _____

DAY 2: Date _____

Morning _____

Midday _____

Evening _____

Snacks _____

___ Meat	___ Bread	___ Vegetable	___ Fruit	___ Milk	___ Fat
☐ Prayer	☐ Bible Study	☐ Scripture Reading	☐ Memory Verse	☐ Encouragement	___ Water

Exercise
Aerobic _____
Strength _____
Flexibility _____

DAY 3: Date _____

Morning _____

Midday _____

Evening _____

Snacks _____

___ Meat	___ Bread	___ Vegetable	___ Fruit	___ Milk	___ Fat
☐ Prayer	☐ Bible Study	☐ Scripture Reading	☐ Memory Verse	☐ Encouragement	___ Water

Exercise
Aerobic _____
Strength _____
Flexibility _____

DAY 4: Date _____

Morning _____

Midday _____

Evening _____

Snacks _____

___ Meat	___ Bread	___ Vegetable	___ Fruit	___ Milk	___ Fat
☐ Prayer	☐ Bible Study	☐ Scripture Reading	☐ Memory Verse	☐ Encouragement	___ Water

Exercise
Aerobic _____
Strength _____
Flexibility _____

Name _____

Date _____ through _____

Week # _____ Calorie Level _____

Daily Exchange Plan

Level	Meat	Bread	Veggie	Fruit	Milk	Fat
1200	4-5	5-6	3	2-3	2-3	3-4
1400	5-6	6-7	3-4	3-4	2-3	3-4
1500	5-6	7-8	3-4	3-4	2-3	3-4
1600	6-7	8-9	3-4	3-4	2-3	3-4
1800	6-7	10-11	3-4	3-4	2-3	4-5
2000	6-7	11-12	4-5	4-5	2-3	4-5
2200	7-8	12-13	4-5	4-5	2-3	6-7
2400	8-9	13-14	4-5	4-5	2-3	7-8
2600	9-10	14-15	5	5	2-3	7-8
2800	9-10	15-16	5	5	2-3	9

You may always choose the high range of vegetables and fruits. Limit your high range selections to only one of the following: meat, bread, milk or fat.

_____ Loss _____ Gain _____ Maintain

_____ Attendance   _____ Bible Study
_____ Prayer   _____ Scripture Reading
_____ Memory Verse   _____ CR
_____ Encouragement
_____ Exercise
Aerobic _____
Strength _____
Flexibility _____

DAY 5: Date _____

Morning _____

Midday _____

Evening _____

Snacks _____

_____ Meat
_____ Bread
_____ Vegetable
_____ Fruit
_____ Milk
_____ Fat

☐ Prayer
☐ Bible Study
☐ Scripture Reading
☐ Memory Verse
☐ Encouragement
_____ Water

Exercise
Aerobic _____
Strength _____
Flexibility _____

DAY 6: Date _____

Morning _____

Midday _____

Evening _____

Snacks _____

_____ Meat
_____ Bread
_____ Vegetable
_____ Fruit
_____ Milk
_____ Fat

☐ Prayer
☐ Bible Study
☐ Scripture Reading
☐ Memory Verse
☐ Encouragement
_____ Water

Exercise
Aerobic _____
Strength _____
Flexibility _____

DAY 7: Date _____

Morning _____

Midday _____

Evening _____

Snacks _____

_____ Meat
_____ Bread
_____ Vegetable
_____ Fruit
_____ Milk
_____ Fat

☐ Prayer
☐ Bible Study
☐ Scripture Reading
☐ Memory Verse
☐ Encouragement
_____ Water

Exercise
Aerobic _____
Strength _____
Flexibility _____

DAY 1: Date _____

Morning _____

Midday _____

Evening _____

Snacks _____

☐ Prayer	☐ Bible Study
___ Meat	☐ Memory Verse
___ Bread	☐ Encouragement
___ Vegetable ___ Scripture Reading	
___ Fruit	
___ Milk	
___ Fat ___ Water	

Exercise
Aerobic _____
Strength _____
Flexibility _____

DAY 2: Date _____

Morning _____

Midday _____

Evening _____

Snacks _____

☐ Prayer	☐ Bible Study
___ Meat	☐ Memory Verse
___ Bread	☐ Encouragement
___ Vegetable ___ Scripture Reading	
___ Fruit	
___ Milk	
___ Fat ___ Water	

Exercise
Aerobic _____
Strength _____
Flexibility _____

DAY 3: Date _____

Morning _____

Midday _____

Evening _____

Snacks _____

☐ Prayer	☐ Bible Study
___ Meat	☐ Memory Verse
___ Bread	☐ Encouragement
___ Vegetable ___ Scripture Reading	
___ Fruit	
___ Milk	
___ Fat ___ Water	

Exercise
Aerobic _____
Strength _____
Flexibility _____

DAY 4: Date _____

Morning _____

Midday _____

Evening _____

Snacks _____

☐ Prayer	☐ Bible Study
___ Meat	☐ Memory Verse
___ Bread	☐ Encouragement
___ Vegetable ___ Scripture Reading	
___ Fruit	
___ Milk	
___ Fat ___ Water	

Exercise
Aerobic _____
Strength _____
Flexibility _____

FIRST PLACE CR

Name _____

Date _____ through _____

Week # _____ Calorie Level _____

Daily Exchange Plan

Level	Meat	Bread	Veggie	Fruit	Milk	Fat
1200	4-5	5-6	3	2-3	2-3	3-4
1400	5-6	6-7	3-4	3-4	2-3	3-4
1500	5-6	7-8	3-4	3-4	2-3	3-4
1600	6-7	8-9	3-4	3-4	2-3	3-4
1800	6-7	10-11	3-4	3-4	2-3	4-5
2000	6-7	11-12	4-5	4-5	2-3	4-5
2200	7-8	12-13	4-5	4-5	2-3	6-7
2400	8-9	13-14	4-5	4-5	2-3	7-8
2600	9-10	14-15	5	5	2-3	7-8
2800	9-10	15-16	5	5	2-3	9

You may always choose the high range of vegetables and fruits. Limit your high range selections to only one of the following: meat, bread, milk or fat.

_____ Loss _____ Gain _____ Maintain

_____ Attendance _____ Bible Study
_____ Prayer _____ Scripture Reading
_____ Memory Verse _____ CR
_____ Encouragement
_____ Exercise
Aerobic _____

Strength _____
Flexibility _____

DAY 5: Date _____

Morning _____

Midday _____

Evening _____

Snacks _____

_____ Meat   ☐ Prayer
_____ Bread   ☐ Bible Study
_____ Vegetable   ☐ Scripture Reading
_____ Fruit   ☐ Memory Verse
_____ Milk   ☐ Encouragement
_____ Fat   _____ Water

Exercise
Aerobic _____

Strength _____
Flexibility _____

DAY 6: Date _____

Morning _____

Midday _____

Evening _____

Snacks _____

_____ Meat   ☐ Prayer
_____ Bread   ☐ Bible Study
_____ Vegetable   ☐ Scripture Reading
_____ Fruit   ☐ Memory Verse
_____ Milk   ☐ Encouragement
_____ Fat   _____ Water

Exercise
Aerobic _____

Strength _____
Flexibility _____

DAY 7: Date _____

Morning _____

Midday _____

Evening _____

Snacks _____

_____ Meat   ☐ Prayer
_____ Bread   ☐ Bible Study
_____ Vegetable   ☐ Scripture Reading
_____ Fruit   ☐ Memory Verse
_____ Milk   ☐ Encouragement
_____ Fat   _____ Water

Exercise
Aerobic _____

Strength _____
Flexibility _____

DAY 1: Date _____

Morning _____

Midday _____

Evening _____

Snacks _____

____ Meat ____	☐ Prayer
____ Bread ____	☐ Bible Study
____ Vegetable ____	☐ Scripture Reading
____ Fruit ____	☐ Memory Verse
____ Milk ____	☐ Encouragement
____ Fat ____	____ Water

Exercise
Aerobic _____
Strength _____
Flexibili.y _____

DAY 2: Date _____

Morning _____

Midday _____

Evening _____

Snacks _____

____ Meat ____	☐ Prayer
____ Bread ____	☐ Bible Study
____ Vegetable ____	☐ Scripture Reading
____ Fruit ____	☐ Memory Verse
____ Milk ____	☐ Encouragement
____ Fat ____	____ Water

Exercise
Aerobic _____
Strength _____
Flexibility _____

DAY 3: Date _____

Morning _____

Midday _____

Evening _____

Snacks _____

____ Meat ____	☐ Prayer
____ Bread ____	☐ Bible Study
____ Vegetable ____	☐ Scripture Reading
____ Fruit ____	☐ Memory Verse
____ Milk ____	☐ Encouragement
____ Fat ____	____ Water

Exercise
Aerobic _____
Strength _____
Flexibility _____

DAY 4: Date _____

Morning _____

Midday _____

Evening _____

Snacks _____

____ Meat ____	☐ Prayer
____ Bread ____	☐ Bible Study
____ Vegetable ____	☐ Scripture Reading
____ Fruit ____	☐ Memory Verse
____ Milk ____	☐ Encouragement
____ Fat ____	____ Water

Exercise
Aerobic _____
Strength _____
Flexibility _____

FIRST PLACE CR

Name _____

Date _____ through _____

Week # _____ Calorie Level _____

Daily Exchange Plan

Level	Meat	Bread	Veggie	Fruit	Milk	Fat
1200	4-5	5-6	3	2-3	2-3	3-4
1400	5-6	6-7	3-4	3-4	2-3	3-4
1500	5-6	7-8	3-4	3-4	2-3	3-4
1600	6-7	8-9	3-4	3-4	2-3	3-4
1800	6-7	10-11	3-4	3-4	2-3	4-5
2000	6-7	11-12	4-5	4-5	2-3	4-5
2200	7-8	12-13	4-5	4-5	2-3	6-7
2400	8-9	13-14	4-5	4-5	2-3	7-8
2600	9-10	14-15	5	5	2-3	7-8
2800	9-10	15-16	5	5	2-3	9

You may always choose the high range of vegetables and fruits. Limit your high range selections to only one of the following: meat, bread, milk or fat.

_____ Loss _____ Gain _____ Maintain

_____ Attendance _____ Bible Study
_____ Prayer _____ Scripture Reading
_____ Memory Verse _____ CR
_____ Encouragement
_____ Exercise
Aerobic _____

Strength _____
Flexibility _____

DAY 5: Date _____

Morning _____

Midday _____

Evening _____

Snacks _____

_____ Meat   ☐ Prayer
_____ Bread   ☐ Bible Study
_____ Vegetable ☐ Scripture Reading
_____ Fruit   ☐ Memory Verse
_____ Milk   ☐ Encouragement
_____ Fat   _____ Water

Exercise
Aerobic _____

Strength _____
Flexibility _____

DAY 6: Date _____

Morning _____

Midday _____

Evening _____

Snacks _____

_____ Meat   ☐ Prayer
_____ Bread   ☐ Bible Study
_____ Vegetable ☐ Scripture Reading
_____ Fruit   ☐ Memory Verse
_____ Milk   ☐ Encouragement
_____ Fat   _____ Water

Exercise
Aerobic _____

Strength _____
Flexibility _____

DAY 7: Date _____

Morning _____

Midday _____

Evening _____

Snacks _____

_____ Meat   ☐ Prayer
_____ Bread   ☐ Bible Study
_____ Vegetable ☐ Scripture Reading
_____ Fruit   ☐ Memory Verse
_____ Milk   ☐ Encouragement
_____ Fat   _____ Water

Exercise
Aerobic _____

Strength _____
Flexibility _____

DAY 1: Date ___

Morning ___

Midday ___

Evening ___

Snacks ___

☐ Prayer	☐ Bible Study
☐ Scripture Reading	☐ Memory Verse
☐ Encouragement	

___ Meat ___ Bread
___ Vegetable ___ Fruit
___ Milk ___ Fat
___ Water

Exercise
Aerobic ___
Strength ___
Flexibility ___

DAY 2: Date ___

Morning ___

Midday ___

Evening ___

Snacks ___

☐ Prayer	☐ Bible Study
☐ Scripture Reading	☐ Memory Verse
☐ Encouragement	

___ Meat ___ Bread
___ Vegetable ___ Fruit
___ Milk ___ Fat
___ Water

Exercise
Aerobic ___
Strength ___
Flexibility ___

DAY 3: Date ___

Morning ___

Midday ___

Evening ___

Snacks ___

☐ Prayer	☐ Bible Study
☐ Scripture Reading	☐ Memory Verse
☐ Encouragement	

___ Meat ___ Bread
___ Vegetable ___ Fruit
___ Milk ___ Fat
___ Water

Exercise
Aerobic ___
Strength ___
Flexibility ___

DAY 4: Date ___

Morning ___

Midday ___

Evening ___

Snacks ___

☐ Prayer	☐ Bible Study
☐ Scripture Reading	☐ Memory Verse
☐ Encouragement	

___ Meat ___ Bread
___ Vegetable ___ Fruit
___ Milk ___ Fat
___ Water

Exercise
Aerobic ___
Strength ___
Flexibility ___

FIRST PLACE CR

Name _____

Date _____ through _____

Week # _____ Calorie Level _____

Daily Exchange Plan

Level	Meat	Bread	Veggie	Fruit	Milk	Fat
1200	4-5	5-6	3	2-3	2-3	3-4
1400	5-6	6-7	3-4	3-4	2-3	3-4
1500	5-6	7-8	3-4	3-4	2-3	3-4
1600	6-7	8-9	3-4	3-4	2-3	3-4
1800	6-7	10-11	3-4	3-4	2-3	4-5
2000	6-7	11-12	4-5	4-5	2-3	4-5
2200	7-8	12-13	4-5	4-5	2-3	6-7
2400	8-9	13-14	4-5	4-5	2-3	7-8
2600	9-10	14-15	5	5	2-3	7-8
2800	9-10	15-16	5	5	2-3	9

You may always choose the high range of vegetables and fruits. Limit your high range selections to only one of the following: meat, bread, milk or fat.

_____ Loss _____ Gain _____ Maintain

_____ Attendance _____ Bible Study
_____ Prayer _____ Scripture Reading
_____ Memory Verse _____ CR
_____ Encouragement
_____ Exercise
_____ Aerobic

_____ Strength
_____ Flexibility

DAY 5: Date _____

Morning _____

Midday _____

Evening _____

Snacks _____

_____ Meat   ☐ Prayer
_____ Bread   ☐ Bible Study
_____ Vegetable   ☐ Scripture Reading
_____ Fruit   ☐ Memory Verse
_____ Milk   ☐ Encouragement
_____ Fat   _____ Water

Exercise _____
Aerobic _____

Strength _____
Flexibility _____

DAY 6: Date _____

Morning _____

Midday _____

Evening _____

Snacks _____

_____ Meat   ☐ Prayer
_____ Bread   ☐ Bible Study
_____ Vegetable   ☐ Scripture Reading
_____ Fruit   ☐ Memory Verse
_____ Milk   ☐ Encouragement
_____ Fat   _____ Water

Exercise _____
Aerobic _____

Strength _____
Flexibility _____

DAY 7: Date _____

Morning _____

Midday _____

Evening _____

Snacks _____

_____ Meat   ☐ Prayer
_____ Bread   ☐ Bible Study
_____ Vegetable   ☐ Scripture Reading
_____ Fruit   ☐ Memory Verse
_____ Milk   ☐ Encouragement
_____ Fat   _____ Water

Exercise _____
Aerobic _____

Strength _____
Flexibility _____

DAY 1: Date _____   **DAY 2:** Date _____   **DAY 3:** Date _____   **DAY 4:** Date _____

Each day contains the same form:

Morning _____

Midday _____

Evening _____

Snacks _____

___ Meat	☐ Prayer
___ Bread	☐ Bible Study
___ Vegetable	☐ Scripture Reading
___ Fruit	☐ Memory Verse
___ Milk	☐ Encouragement
___ Fat	___ Water

Exercise

Aerobic _____

Strength _____

Flexibility _____

FIRST PLACE CR

Name _____

Date _____ through _____

Week # _____ Calorie Level _____

Daily Exchange Plan

Level	Meat	Bread	Veggie	Fruit	Milk	Fat
1200	4-5	5-6	3	2-3	2-3	3-4
1400	5-6	6-7	3-4	3-4	2-3	3-4
1500	5-6	7-8	3-4	3-4	2-3	3-4
1600	6-7	8-9	3-4	3-4	2-3	3-4
1800	6-7	10-11	3-4	3-4	2-3	4-5
2000	6-7	11-12	4-5	4-5	2-3	4-5
2200	7-8	12-13	4-5	4-5	2-3	6-7
2400	8-9	13-14	4-5	4-5	2-3	7-8
2600	9-10	14-15	5	5	2-3	7-8
2800	9-10	15-16	5	5	2-3	9

You may always choose the high range of vegetables and fruits. Limit your high range selections to only one of the following: meat, bread, milk or fat.

_____ Loss _____ Gain _____ Maintain

_____ Attendance   _____ Bible Study
_____ Prayer   _____ Scripture Reading
_____ Memory Verse _____ CR
_____ Encouragement
_____ Exercise
Aerobic _____

Strength _____
Flexibility _____

DAY 5: Date _____

Morning _____
_____

Midday _____
_____

Evening _____
_____

Snacks _____
_____

_____ Meat   ☐ Prayer
_____ Bread   ☐ Bible Study
_____ Vegetable   ☐ Scripture Reading
_____ Fruit   ☐ Memory Verse
_____ Milk   ☐ Encouragement
_____ Fat   Water _____

Exercise
Aerobic _____

Strength _____
Flexibility _____

DAY 6: Date _____

Morning _____
_____

Midday _____
_____

Evening _____
_____

Snacks _____
_____

_____ Meat   ☐ Prayer
_____ Bread   ☐ Bible Study
_____ Vegetable   ☐ Scripture Reading
_____ Fruit   ☐ Memory Verse
_____ Milk   ☐ Encouragement
_____ Fat   Water _____

Exercise
Aerobic _____

Strength _____
Flexibility _____

DAY 7: Date _____

Morning _____
_____

Midday _____
_____

Evening _____
_____

Snacks _____
_____

_____ Meat   ☐ Prayer
_____ Bread   ☐ Bible Study
_____ Vegetable   ☐ Scripture Reading
_____ Fruit   ☐ Memory Verse
_____ Milk   ☐ Encouragement
_____ Fat   Water _____

Exercise
Aerobic _____

Strength _____
Flexibility _____

DAY 1: Date _____

Morning _____

Midday _____

Evening _____

Snacks _____

___ Meat   ☐ Prayer
___ Bread   ☐ Bible Study
___ Vegetable   ☐ Scripture Reading
___ Fruit   ☐ Memory Verse
___ Milk   ☐ Encouragement
___ Fat   ___ Water

Exercise
Aerobic _____
Strength _____
Flexibility _____

DAY 2: Date _____

Morning _____

Midday _____

Evening _____

Snacks _____

___ Meat   ☐ Prayer
___ Bread   ☐ Bible Study
___ Vegetable   ☐ Scripture Reading
___ Fruit   ☐ Memory Verse
___ Milk   ☐ Encouragement
___ Fat   ___ Water

Exercise
Aerobic _____
Strength _____
Flexibility _____

DAY 3: Date _____

Morning _____

Midday _____

Evening _____

Snacks _____

___ Meat   ☐ Prayer
___ Bread   ☐ Bible Study
___ Vegetable   ☐ Scripture Reading
___ Fruit   ☐ Memory Verse
___ Milk   ☐ Encouragement
___ Fat   ___ Water

Exercise
Aerobic _____
Strength _____
Flexibility _____

DAY 4: Date _____

Morning _____

Midday _____

Evening _____

Snacks _____

___ Meat   ☐ Prayer
___ Bread   ☐ Bible Study
___ Vegetable   ☐ Scripture Reading
___ Fruit   ☐ Memory Verse
___ Milk   ☐ Encouragement
___ Fat   ___ Water

Exercise
Aerobic _____
Strength _____
Flexibility _____

FIRST PLACE CR

Name _____

Date _____ through _____

Week # _____ Calorie Level _____

Daily Exchange Plan

Level	Meat	Bread	Veggie	Fruit	Milk	Fat
1200	4-5	5-6	3	2-3	2-3	3-4
1400	5-6	6-7	3-4	3-4	2-3	3-4
1500	5-6	7-8	3-4	3-4	2-3	3-4
1600	6-7	8-9	3-4	3-4	2-3	3-4
1800	6-7	10-11	3-4	3-4	2-3	4-5
2000	6-7	11-12	4-5	4-5	2-3	4-5
2200	7-8	12-13	4-5	4-5	2-3	6-7
2400	8-9	13-14	4-5	4-5	2-3	7-8
2600	9-10	14-15	5	5	2-3	7-8
2800	9-10	15-16	5	5	2-3	9

You may always choose the high range of vegetables and fruits. Limit your high range selections to only one of the following: meat, bread, milk or fat.

_____ Loss _____ Gain _____ Maintain

_____ Attendance _____ Bible Study
_____ Prayer _____ Scripture Reading
_____ Memory Verse _____ CR
_____ Encouragement
_____ Exercise
Aerobic _____
Strength _____
Flexibility _____

DAY 5: Date _____

Morning _____

Midday _____

Evening _____

Snacks _____

_____ Meat   ☐ Prayer
_____ Bread   ☐ Bible Study
_____ Vegetable   ☐ Scripture Reading
_____ Fruit   ☐ Memory Verse
_____ Milk   ☐ Encouragement
_____ Fat   Water _____

Exercise
Aerobic _____

Strength _____
Flexibility _____

DAY 6: Date _____

Morning _____

Midday _____

Evening _____

Snacks _____

_____ Meat   ☐ Prayer
_____ Bread   ☐ Bible Study
_____ Vegetable   ☐ Scripture Reading
_____ Fruit   ☐ Memory Verse
_____ Milk   ☐ Encouragement
_____ Fat   Water _____

Exercise
Aerobic _____

Strength _____
Flexibility _____

DAY 7: Date _____

Morning _____

Midday _____

Evening _____

Snacks _____

_____ Meat   ☐ Prayer
_____ Bread   ☐ Bible Study
_____ Vegetable   ☐ Scripture Reading
_____ Fruit   ☐ Memory Verse
_____ Milk   ☐ Encouragement
_____ Fat   Water _____

Exercise
Aerobic _____

Strength _____
Flexibility _____

DAY 1: Date _____

Morning _____

Midday _____

Evening _____

Snacks _____

- ☐ Prayer
- ☐ Bible Study
- ☐ Scripture Reading
- ☐ Memory Verse
- ☐ Encouragement

_____ Meat
_____ Bread
_____ Vegetable
_____ Fruit
_____ Milk
_____ Fat
_____ Water

Exercise
Aerobic _____
Strength _____
Flexibility _____

DAY 2: Date _____

Morning _____

Midday _____

Evening _____

Snacks _____

- ☐ Prayer
- ☐ Bible Study
- ☐ Scripture Reading
- ☐ Memory Verse
- ☐ Encouragement

_____ Meat
_____ Bread
_____ Vegetable
_____ Fruit
_____ Milk
_____ Fat
_____ Water

Exercise
Aerobic _____
Strength _____
Flexibility _____

DAY 3: Date _____

Morning _____

Midday _____

Evening _____

Snacks _____

- ☐ Prayer
- ☐ Bible Study
- ☐ Scripture Reading
- ☐ Memory Verse
- ☐ Encouragement

_____ Meat
_____ Bread
_____ Vegetable
_____ Fruit
_____ Milk
_____ Fat
_____ Water

Exercise
Aerobic _____
Strength _____
Flexibility _____

DAY 4: Date _____

Morning _____

Midday _____

Evening _____

Snacks _____

- ☐ Prayer
- ☐ Bible Study
- ☐ Scripture Reading
- ☐ Memory Verse
- ☐ Encouragement

_____ Meat
_____ Bread
_____ Vegetable
_____ Fruit
_____ Milk
_____ Fat
_____ Water

Exercise
Aerobic _____
Strength _____
Flexibility _____

Name _____

Date _____ through _____

Week # _____ Calorie Level _____

Daily Exchange Plan

Level	Meat	Bread	Veggie	Fruit	Milk	Fat
1200	4-5	5-6	3	2-3	2-3	3-4
1400	5-6	6-7	3-4	3-4	2-3	3-4
1500	5-6	7-8	3-4	3-4	2-3	3-4
1600	6-7	8-9	3-4	3-4	2-3	3-4
1800	6-7	10-11	3-4	3-4	2-3	4-5
2000	6-7	11-12	4-5	4-5	2-3	4-5
2200	7-8	12-13	4-5	4-5	2-3	6-7
2400	8-9	13-14	4-5	4-5	2-3	7-8
2600	9-10	14-15	5	5	2-3	7-8
2800	9-10	15-16	5	5	2-3	9

You may always choose the high range of vegetables and fruits. Limit your high range selections to only one of the following: meat, bread, milk or fat.

_____ Loss _____ Gain _____ Maintain

_____ Attendance _____ Bible Study
_____ Prayer _____ Scripture Reading
_____ Memory Verse _____ CR
_____ Encouragement
_____ Exercise
Aerobic _____

Strength _____
Flexibility _____

DAY 5: Date _____

Morning _____

Midday _____

Evening _____

Snacks _____

_____ Meat   ☐ Prayer
_____ Bread   ☐ Bible Study
_____ Vegetable ☐ Scripture Reading
_____ Fruit   ☐ Memory Verse
_____ Milk   ☐ Encouragement
_____ Fat   Water _____

Exercise
Aerobic _____

Strength _____
Flexibility _____

DAY 6: Date _____

Morning _____

Midday _____

Evening _____

Snacks _____

_____ Meat   ☐ Prayer
_____ Bread   ☐ Bible Study
_____ Vegetable ☐ Scripture Reading
_____ Fruit   ☐ Memory Verse
_____ Milk   ☐ Encouragement
_____ Fat   Water _____

Exercise
Aerobic _____

Strength _____
Flexibility _____

DAY 7: Date _____

Morning _____

Midday _____

Evening _____

Snacks _____

_____ Meat   ☐ Prayer
_____ Bread   ☐ Bible Study
_____ Vegetable ☐ Scripture Reading
_____ Fruit   ☐ Memory Verse
_____ Milk   ☐ Encouragement
_____ Fat   Water _____

Exercise
Aerobic _____

Strength _____
Flexibility _____

DAY 1: Date _____

Morning _____

Midday _____

Evening _____

Snacks _____

___ Meat	☐ Prayer
___ Bread	☐ Bible Study
___ Vegetable	☐ Scripture Reading
___ Fruit	☐ Memory Verse
___ Milk	☐ Encouragement
___ Fat	___ Water

Exercise
Aerobic _____
Strength _____
Flexibility _____

DAY 2: Date _____

Morning _____

Midday _____

Evening _____

Snacks _____

___ Meat	☐ Prayer
___ Bread	☐ Bible Study
___ Vegetable	☐ Scripture Reading
___ Fruit	☐ Memory Verse
___ Milk	☐ Encouragement
___ Fat	___ Water

Exercise
Aerobic _____
Strength _____
Flexibility _____

DAY 3: Date _____

Morning _____

Midday _____

Evening _____

Snacks _____

___ Meat	☐ Prayer
___ Bread	☐ Bible Study
___ Vegetable	☐ Scripture Reading
___ Fruit	☐ Memory Verse
___ Milk	☐ Encouragement
___ Fat	___ Water

Exercise
Aerobic _____
Strength _____
Flexibility _____

DAY 4: Date _____

Morning _____

Midday _____

Evening _____

Snacks _____

___ Meat	☐ Prayer
___ Bread	☐ Bible Study
___ Vegetable	☐ Scripture Reading
___ Fruit	☐ Memory Verse
___ Milk	☐ Encouragement
___ Fat	___ Water

Exercise
Aerobic _____
Strength _____
Flexibility _____

FIRST PLACE CR

Name _____

Date _____ through _____

Week # _____ Calorie Level _____

Daily Exchange Plan

Level	Meat	Bread	Veggie	Fruit	Milk	Fat
1200	4-5	5-6	3	2-3	2-3	3-4
1400	5-6	6-7	3-4	3-4	2-3	3-4
1500	5-6	7-8	3-4	3-4	2-3	3-4
1600	6-7	8-9	3-4	3-4	2-3	3-4
1800	6-7	10-11	3-4	3-4	2-3	4-5
2000	6-7	11-12	4-5	4-5	2-3	4-5
2200	7-8	12-13	4-5	4-5	2-3	6-7
2400	8-9	13-14	4-5	4-5	2-3	7-8
2600	9-10	14-15	5	5	2-3	7-8
2800	9-10	15-16	5	5	2-3	9

You may always choose the high range of vegetables and fruits. Limit your high range selections to only one of the following: meat, bread, milk or fat.

___ Loss ___ Gain ___ Maintain

___ Attendance ___ Bible Study
___ Prayer ___ Scripture Reading
___ Memory Verse ___ CR
___ Encouragement
___ Exercise
Aerobic _____

Strength _____
Flexibility _____

DAY 5: Date _____

Morning _____

Midday _____

Evening _____

Snacks _____

___ Meat   ☐ Prayer
___ Bread   ☐ Bible Study
___ Vegetable   ☐ Scripture Reading
___ Fruit   ☐ Memory Verse
___ Milk   ☐ Encouragement
___ Fat   ___ Water

Exercise
Aerobic _____

Strength _____
Flexibility _____

DAY 6: Date _____

Morning _____

Midday _____

Evening _____

Snacks _____

___ Meat   ☐ Prayer
___ Bread   ☐ Bible Study
___ Vegetable   ☐ Scripture Reading
___ Fruit   ☐ Memory Verse
___ Milk   ☐ Encouragement
___ Fat   ___ Water

Exercise
Aerobic _____

Strength _____
Flexibility _____

DAY 7: Date _____

Morning _____

Midday _____

Evening _____

Snacks _____

___ Meat   ☐ Prayer
___ Bread   ☐ Bible Study
___ Vegetable   ☐ Scripture Reading
___ Fruit   ☐ Memory Verse
___ Milk   ☐ Encouragement
___ Fat   ___ Water

Exercise
Aerobic _____

Strength _____
Flexibility _____

DAY 1: Date _____

Morning _____

Midday _____

Evening _____

Snacks _____

___ Meat	☐ Prayer
___ Bread	☐ Bible Study
___ Vegetable	☐ Scripture Reading
___ Fruit	☐ Memory Verse
___ Milk	☐ Encouragement
___ Fat	___ Water

Exercise
Aerobic _____
Strength _____
Flexibility _____

DAY 2: Date _____

Morning _____

Midday _____

Evening _____

Snacks _____

___ Meat	☐ Prayer
___ Bread	☐ Bible Study
___ Vegetable	☐ Scripture Reading
___ Fruit	☐ Memory Verse
___ Milk	☐ Encouragement
___ Fat	___ Water

Exercise
Aerobic _____
Strength _____
Flexibility _____

DAY 3: Date _____

Morning _____

Midday _____

Evening _____

Snacks _____

___ Meat	☐ Prayer
___ Bread	☐ Bible Study
___ Vegetable	☐ Scripture Reading
___ Fruit	☐ Memory Verse
___ Milk	☐ Encouragement
___ Fat	___ Water

Exercise
Aerobic _____
Strength _____
Flexibility _____

DAY 4: Date _____

Morning _____

Midday _____

Evening _____

Snacks _____

___ Meat	☐ Prayer
___ Bread	☐ Bible Study
___ Vegetable	☐ Scripture Reading
___ Fruit	☐ Memory Verse
___ Milk	☐ Encouragement
___ Fat	___ Water

Exercise
Aerobic _____
Strength _____
Flexibility _____

FIRST PLACE CR

Name _____

Date _____ through _____

Week # _____ Calorie Level _____

Daily Exchange Plan

Level	Meat	Bread	Veggie	Fruit	Milk	Fat
1200	4-5	5-6	3	2-3	2-3	3-4
1400	5-6	6-7	3-4	3-4	2-3	3-4
1500	5-6	7-8	3-4	3-4	2-3	3-4
1600	6-7	8-9	3-4	3-4	2-3	3-4
1800	6-7	10-11	3-4	3-4	2-3	4-5
2000	6-7	11-12	4-5	4-5	2-3	4-5
2200	7-8	12-13	4-5	4-5	2-3	6-7
2400	8-9	13-14	4-5	4-5	2-3	7-8
2600	9-10	14-15	5	5	2-3	7-8
2800	9-10	15-16	5	5	2-3	9

You may always choose the high range of vegetables and fruits. Limit your high range selections to only one of the following: meat, bread, milk or fat.

_____ Loss _____ Gain _____ Maintain

_____ Attendance _____ Bible Study
_____ Prayer _____ Scripture Reading
_____ Memory Verse _____ CR
_____ Encouragement
_____ Exercise
Aerobic _____

Strength _____
Flexibility _____

DAY 5: Date _____

Morning _____

Midday _____

Evening _____

Snacks _____

_____ Meat ☐ Prayer
_____ Bread ☐ Bible Study
_____ Vegetable ☐ Scripture Reading
_____ Fruit ☐ Memory Verse
_____ Milk ☐ Encouragement
_____ Fat ☐ Water

Exercise
Aerobic _____

Strength _____
Flexibility _____

DAY 6: Date _____

Morning _____

Midday _____

Evening _____

Snacks _____

_____ Meat ☐ Prayer
_____ Bread ☐ Bible Study
_____ Vegetable ☐ Scripture Reading
_____ Fruit ☐ Memory Verse
_____ Milk ☐ Encouragement
_____ Fat ☐ Water

Exercise
Aerobic _____

Strength _____
Flexibility _____

DAY 7: Date _____

Morning _____

Midday _____

Evening _____

Snacks _____

_____ Meat ☐ Prayer
_____ Bread ☐ Bible Study
_____ Vegetable ☐ Scripture Reading
_____ Fruit ☐ Memory Verse
_____ Milk ☐ Encouragement
_____ Fat ☐ Water

Exercise
Aerobic _____

Strength _____
Flexibility _____

DAY 1: Date _____

Morning _____

Midday _____

Evening _____

Snacks _____

___ Meat   □ Prayer
___ Bread   □ Bible Study
___ Vegetable   □ Scripture Reading
___ Fruit   □ Memory Verse
___ Milk   □ Encouragement
___ Fat   ___ Water

Exercise
Aerobic _____
Strength _____
Flexibility _____

DAY 2: Date _____

Morning _____

Midday _____

Evening _____

Snacks _____

___ Meat   □ Prayer
___ Bread   □ Bible Study
___ Vegetable   □ Scripture Reading
___ Fruit   □ Memory Verse
___ Milk   □ Encouragement
___ Fat   ___ Water

Exercise
Aerobic _____
Strength _____
Flexibility _____

DAY 3: Date _____

Morning _____

Midday _____

Evening _____

Snacks _____

___ Meat   □ Prayer
___ Bread   □ Bible Study
___ Vegetable   □ Scripture Reading
___ Fruit   □ Memory Verse
___ Milk   □ Encouragement
___ Fat   ___ Water

Exercise
Aerobic _____
Strength _____
Flexibility _____

DAY 4: Date _____

Morning _____

Midday _____

Evening _____

Snacks _____

___ Meat   □ Prayer
___ Bread   □ Bible Study
___ Vegetable   □ Scripture Reading
___ Fruit   □ Memory Verse
___ Milk   □ Encouragement
___ Fat   ___ Water

Exercise
Aerobic _____
Strength _____
Flexibility _____

FIRST PLACE CR

Name _____

Date _____ through _____

Week # _____ Calorie Level _____

Daily Exchange Plan

Level	Meat	Bread	Veggie	Fruit	Milk	Fat
1200	4-5	5-6	3	2-3	2-3	3-4
1400	5-6	6-7	3-4	3-4	2-3	3-4
1500	5-6	7-8	3-4	3-4	2-3	3-4
1600	6-7	8-9	3-4	3-4	2-3	3-4
1800	6-7	10-11	3-4	3-4	2-3	4-5
2000	6-7	11-12	4-5	4-5	2-3	4-5
2200	7-8	12-13	4-5	4-5	2-3	6-7
2400	8-9	13-14	4-5	4-5	2-3	7-8
2600	9-10	14-15	5	5	2-3	7-8
2800	9-10	15-16	5	5	2-3	9

You may always choose the high range of vegetables and fruits. Limit your high range selections to only one of the following: meat, bread, milk or fat.

_____ Loss _____ Gain _____ Maintain

_____ Attendance _____ Bible Study
_____ Prayer _____ Scripture Reading
_____ Memory Verse _____ CR
_____ Encouragement
_____ Exercise

Aerobic _____

Strength _____
Flexibility _____

DAY 5: Date _____

Morning _____

Midday _____

Evening _____

Snacks _____

_____ Meat   ☐ Prayer
_____ Bread   ☐ Bible Study
_____ Vegetable   ☐ Scripture Reading
_____ Fruit   ☐ Memory Verse
_____ Milk   ☐ Encouragement
_____ Fat   _____ Water

Exercise _____
Aerobic _____

Strength _____
Flexibility _____

DAY 6: Date _____

Morning _____

Midday _____

Evening _____

Snacks _____

_____ Meat   ☐ Prayer
_____ Bread   ☐ Bible Study
_____ Vegetable   ☐ Scripture Reading
_____ Fruit   ☐ Memory Verse
_____ Milk   ☐ Encouragement
_____ Fat   _____ Water

Exercise _____
Aerobic _____

Strength _____
Flexibility _____

DAY 7: Date _____

Morning _____

Midday _____

Evening _____

Snacks _____

_____ Meat   ☐ Prayer
_____ Bread   ☐ Bible Study
_____ Vegetable   ☐ Scripture Reading
_____ Fruit   ☐ Memory Verse
_____ Milk   ☐ Encouragement
_____ Fat   _____ Water

Exercise _____
Aerobic _____

Strength _____
Flexibility _____

DAY 1: Date _____

Morning _____

Midday _____

Evening _____

Snacks _____

___ Meat	☐ Prayer
___ Bread	☐ Bible Study
___ Vegetable	☐ Scripture Reading
___ Fruit	☐ Memory Verse
___ Milk	☐ Encouragement
___ Fat ___ Water	

Exercise
Aerobic _____
Strength _____
Flexibility _____

DAY 2: Date _____

Morning _____

Midday _____

Evening _____

Snacks _____

___ Meat	☐ Prayer
___ Bread	☐ Bible Study
___ Vegetable	☐ Scripture Reading
___ Fruit	☐ Memory Verse
___ Milk	☐ Encouragement
___ Fat ___ Water	

Exercise
Aerobic _____
Strength _____
Flexibility _____

DAY 3: Date _____

Morning _____

Midday _____

Evening _____

Snacks _____

___ Meat	☐ Prayer
___ Bread	☐ Bible Study
___ Vegetable	☐ Scripture Reading
___ Fruit	☐ Memory Verse
___ Milk	☐ Encouragement
___ Fat ___ Water	

Exercise
Aerobic _____
Strength _____
Flexibility _____

DAY 4: Date _____

Morning _____

Midday _____

Evening _____

Snacks _____

___ Meat	☐ Prayer
___ Bread	☐ Bible Study
___ Vegetable	☐ Scripture Reading
___ Fruit	☐ Memory Verse
___ Milk	☐ Encouragement
___ Fat ___ Water	

Exercise
Aerobic _____
Strength _____
Flexibility _____

CONTRIBUTORS

Jody Wilkinson, M.D., M.S., the writer of the Wellness Worksheets for this study, is a physician and exercise physiologist at the Cooper Institute in Dallas, Texas. He trained at the University of Texas Health Science Center in San Antonio, Texas, and Baylor University Medical Center in Dallas. Dr. Wilkinson conducts research on physical activity, nutrition and weight management and has worked with the American Heart Association to develop a health program. He believes strongly in using biblical teaching to motivate people to take care of their physical bodies and enjoy abundant living. Jody and his wife, Natalie, have been married 10 years and have two daughters, Jordan and Sarah, and twin sons, Joel and Cooper.

Scott Wilson, C.E.C., A.A.C., the author of the menu plans in this study, has been cooking professionally for over 20 years. A certified executive chef with the American Culinary Federation, he currently works in the Greater Atlanta area as a personal chef and food consultant and is certified with the United States Personal Chef Associaton. Along with serving as the national food consultant for First Place, he is on the Culinary Program Advisory Board of the Art Institute of Atlanta. Scott has also authored two cookbooks, *Dining Under the Magnolia* and *Healthy Home Cooking*. In his spare time, he is active in church work and spends time with his wife, Jennifer, and their daughter, Katie.

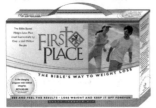

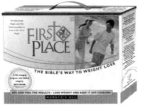

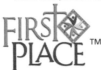
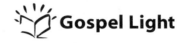